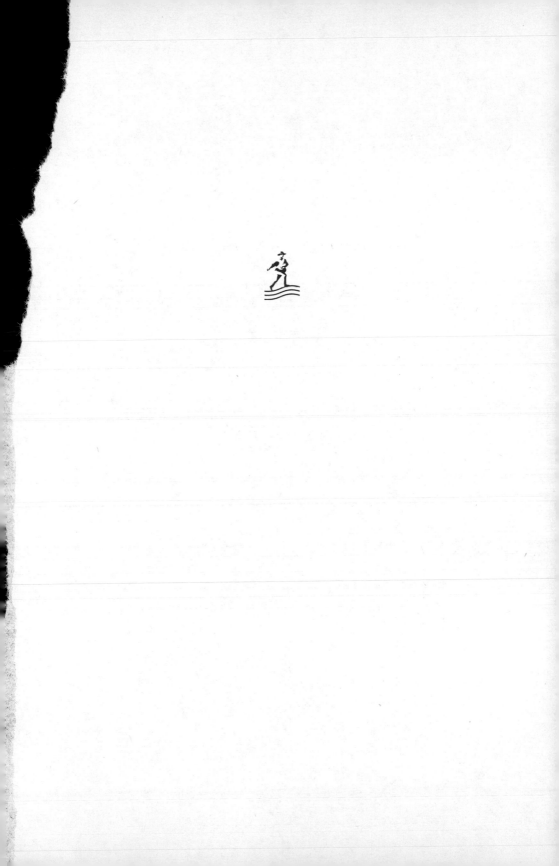

TWO HOURS

The Quest to Run the Impossible Marathon

ED CAESAR

SIMON & SCHUSTER

New York London Toronto Sydney New Delhi

Simon & Schuster
1230 Avenue of the Americas
New York, NY 10020

First Simon & Schuster hardcover edition October 2015

SIMON & SCHUSTER and colophon are registered trademarks of Simon & Schuster, Inc.

For information about special discounts for bulk purchases, please contact Simon & Schuster Special Sales at 1-866-506-1949 or business@simonandschuster.com.

The Simon & Schuster Speakers Bureau can bring authors to your live event. For more information or to book an event contact the Simon & Schuster Speakers Bureau at 1-866-248-3049 or visit our website at www.simonspeakers.com.

Map copyright © 2015 by Jeffrey L. Ward

Manufactured in the United States of America

1   3   5   7   9   10   8   6   4   2

Library of Congress Cataloging-in-Publication Data
Caesar, Ed.
Two hours : the quest to run the impossible marathon / Ed Caesar.—First Simon & Schuster hardcover edition.
        pages cm
1. Marathon running. 2. Marathon running—Training. I. Title.
GV1065.C34 2015
796.42'52—dc23
2014043224

ISBN 978-1-4516-8584-8
ISBN 978-1-4516-8586-2 (ebook)

For Chloë

There is a tide in the affairs of men,
Which, taken at the flood, leads on to fortune;
Omitted, all the voyage of their life
Is bound in shallows and in miseries.
On such a full sea are we now afloat,
And we must take the current when it serves,
Or lose our ventures.

—WILLIAM SHAKESPEARE, *Julius Caesar*

Contents

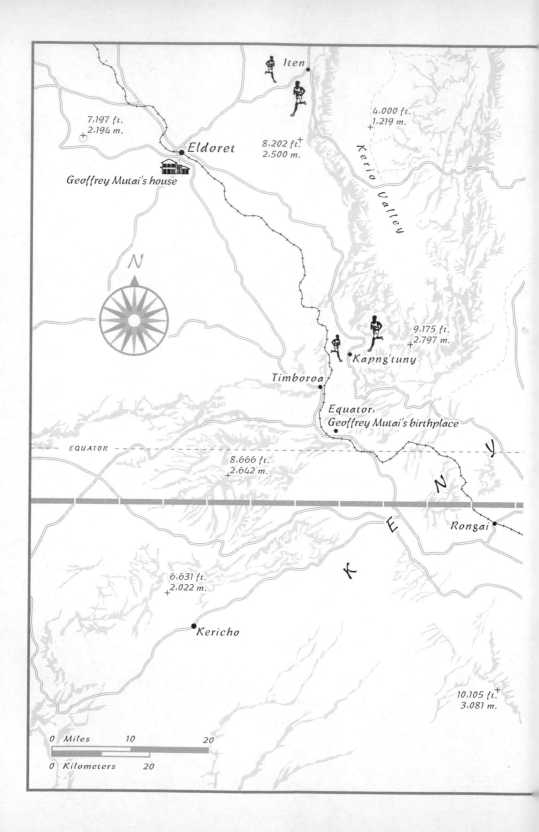

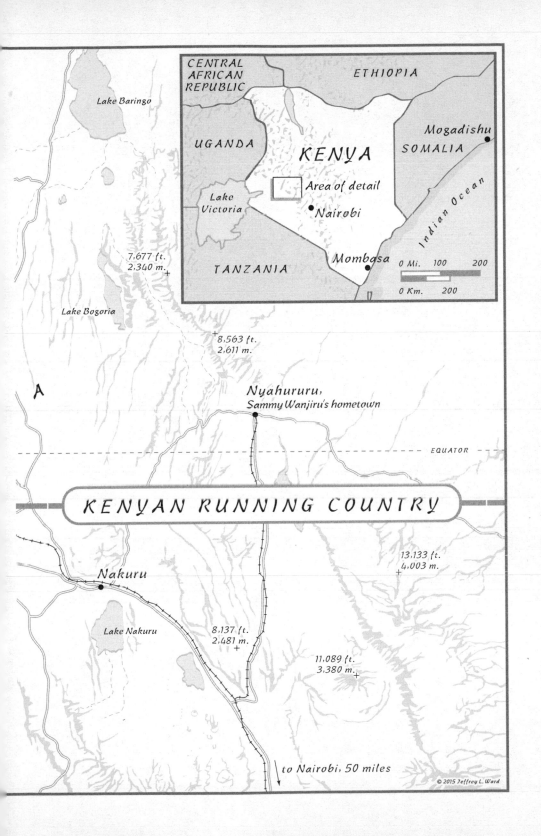

Chapter One

Tear Down This Wall

September 2012

S HORTLY BEFORE nine on a bright fall morning in Berlin, Geoffrey Kiprono Mutai prepared to run a marathon faster than any human being—even he—had run before. A wild, audacious proposition, to propel one's body to such a ragged extreme, and he felt the walls of his quest closing in on him. Years of pain for this one opportunity. Competing voices crowding his head. The loudest saying, *If only we could start running!*

Mutai is five feet seven inches tall, and 125 pounds. He has a wide, expressive face, with a high forehead, elfin ears, and long, gleaming teeth. Most often, you find him amiable, amused, desirous of news and gossip, a flashy smile close by. But now, at this solemn moment, he looked as vulnerable as a foundling.

There were around 41,000 runners behind him. Penned together, they bobbed and lilted like a gentle sea against a harbor wall. Alongside Mutai at the head of the crowd, meanwhile, were two dozen professional athletes whose lives—like his—would be marked irrevocably by the minutes to come. As Mutai ran his final warm-up shuttles, the goosebumps on his chest were visible behind his blood-orange running vest: nerves, or the cold, or both.

Mutai attempted to relieve the tension by telling himself that he didn't need to win the race, or make history, to be happy. *Anywhere on the podium would be okay,* this reasonable voice said. *The marathon is tough. Anything can happen.*

He knew he was fooling himself. It was true, yes, anything could happen in a marathon, and there were many events seemingly outside an athlete's control—including the body's reaction to the stress of racing. No athlete, not even a champion, could know when a cramp or an injury might destroy his chances. So Mutai told himself this thin truth—that his effort was enough. Although he knew that nothing but triumph could satisfy him, and even triumph might not suffice, the mental evasion somehow helped him relax. He needed to relax. Tense legs, he knew, couldn't move.

Mutai said his habitual prayers. For clemency. For strength and for courage. For his stringy legs, veterans and repositories of tens of thousands of miles of training, to carry him another 26 miles and 385 yards. But not for a miracle. He would never ask God for a miracle.

Smiles all around him now: the effervescence of expectation. Mutai could not help but smile too. Despite longing for the starter's pistol, there would always be a part of him that enjoyed these rich, electrified seconds—the warrior part. He was about to race. Yes, the eyes of the city, and the sport, were upon him.

But where else would he want to be? He would shortly express the purest version of his being on the grandest stage imaginable, without saying a word. If the race proceeded as he had dreamed it, he would become not only the world record holder, but a vindicated man. All in a little more than two hours.

———

Mutai is a Kenyan, a Kalenjin, and a Kipsigis. He was born in the village of Equator, which sits at nearly 9,000 feet in the lush highlands at the western escarpment of the Rift Valley, and, as its name suggests, at the beltline of the world. He is a husband, a father, a son, a grandson, a nephew, a cousin, a coach, a businessman, and a potentate. He is a rich man who grew up without shoes.

As the minutes became seconds, and he toed the Berlin startline in his featherweight Adidas racing flats, he was aware that dozens of less successful athletes depended on him for clothes, accommodation, and transport. He knew his family relied on him for their houses, their food, their televisions, their children's school fees, and their cars. He also knew that in this race, he had the chance not only to win 40,000 euros for first place and a possible 80,000 euros in time bonuses (30,000 euros for a time under 2:04:30; 50,000 more for a new world record), but also, if he won in Berlin, the chance to seal a $500,000 jackpot for winning the cumulative World Marathon Majors prize for 2011–2012. And that was just from the organizers of the marathon. His sponsor, Adidas, would also kick in bonuses if he won or became the new world record holder. After agent's fees, he could be more than half a million dollars richer by lunchtime. Back home, his friends and family would be huddled around televisions, watching.

In these final moments of stillness, however, Mutai banished impure thoughts and the crowding, conflicted voices. He attempted to focus. Psychologists talk about a Zen-like state of instinctual action in which the greatest sporting performances are attained. They call it Flow. The French cyclist Jean Bobet described a similar but distinct experience called *La Volupté*, which "is delicate, intimate and ephemeral. It arrives, it takes hold of you, sweeps you up and then leaves you again. It is for you alone. It is a combination of speed and ease, force and grace. It is pure happiness."

Mutai has his own term: the Spirit. The way he understood it, the brutality of his training regime—125 fierce miles a week—was endured to attain this sensation. Thousands of hours of suffering for these minutes of sweetness: speed and ease, force and grace. *The more harder you train,* he would say, *the more you get the Spirit. . . . It* gains *on you.* So far, in his career, the Spirit had allowed Mutai the courage to remake the sport of marathon running, and to destroy previous conceptions of what was possible; to lose his own fear, and implant it in the hearts of his competitors.

Now, on this bright cold day in Berlin, he wished to upend the marathon world once more. As he stood at the head of the vast herd, high banks of loudspeakers began to play the kind of jangling, electronic string music you hear on game shows before the host tells a contestant whether he's landed the big prize. Over these shifting arpeggios came the sound of a stout man with a microphone, counting down the final seconds before the gun. *Ten!* he shouted, in English. *Nine! Eight! Seven . . .* Mutai stood still, his chest pushed forward in anticipation of movement. At that instant, the world receded. Mutai became the instrument of a single imperative—to run a marathon in less than two hours and three minutes.

—

Nine a.m. The gun.

The crowd cheered as thousands of electric-blue balloons were released into the air. The lead athletes shot off and quickly assembled themselves into a group. Within a few hundred meters, these contenders tucked in behind the four elite pacemakers, wearing black-and-white striped vests to distinguish themselves, who in turn followed a BMW on which a digital display was mounted, showing both the elapsed time and the split time for the last kilometer.

In that first group along with Mutai were a handful of extraordinary athletes. Dennis Kimetto had been "discovered" by Mutai in 2008 and now trained in the same group. Nicknamed "Mwafrica," or "the African," by his fellow athletes on account of his coal-black skin, he had progressed rapidly—breaking the 25km world record earlier in 2012—and was now running his first marathon outside Kenya. Geoffrey Kipsang Kamworor, meanwhile, was widely considered to possess a profound natural talent. And, although the nineteen-year-old former junior world cross-country champion was also running his full-marathon debut, he had some experience of Berlin. The previous year, he had paced Haile Gebrselassie, the Ethiopian who is considered by many to be the greatest distance runner of all time, in the race. Haile was so impressed with Kamworor's performance that day that he made an instant prediction: the young Kenyan would one day break the world record himself. And then there was Jonathan Maiyo, who had run a 2:04:56 marathon and a 59:02 half marathon earlier in the year, both world-class times.

Within a couple of kilometers, after the adrenaline burst of the opening section faded, Mutai once again felt freighted with pressure. As the star man in the race, he believed—correctly—that the eyes of his fellow athletes were upon him. If he pushed, he thought, they would push. If he slowed, they would slow. He tried to relax. He prayed again. *God, you know I am fighting. Lead me to the end of the race.* He attempted to put his competitors out of his mind and concentrate on the workings of his own body.

Of the contenders in Berlin, Geoffrey Kamworor (who, like Geoffrey Mutai, pronounces his Christian name "Jo-ffrey") has the most idiosyncratic style. He is powerfully built by marathon runner standards, and has a wide, gap-toothed grin. In training, he looks like a bull before a matador. He runs with one shoulder tucked in and his legs flying straight out behind him. At the dusty athletics track at Chepkoilel, near Eldoret, he leans into tight bends shoulder-first, explosions of orange dust bursting behind him like airstrikes in the desert. Kimetto and Maiyo run more upright. But, while Kimetto's straight back can make him look rigid and uncomfortable, Maiyo's gives him a regal bearing.

Geoffrey Mutai is a paragon of economy. A high-definition, slow-motion camera was once trained on him from a side angle at mile 21 of the 2011 New York City Marathon. At that moment in the race, Mutai was running a 4:31 mile, which is under a two-hour marathon pace. The resulting footage, which is nine seconds long, and available for all to see on the Internet, is hypnotic, and beautiful. Mutai's speed is maintained by a series of sharp midfoot strikes. He doesn't brake at all, or strain for forward movement. There is no tension in his arms. It's as if he is on wheels, not legs.

Watching Mutai in the flesh, head-on and in real time, is no less pleasurable. He runs splay-footed, low-hipped, each stride working the most out of his sinuous calves, while his torso remains as still as a rifle target. Because of this impeccable form, it's sometimes hard to tell when he decides to push the pace. Only the speed of his turnover and the attitude of his head—cast down and bent forward as if at the prow of a clipper—betray his intentions.

———

The official marathon world record on the morning of September 29, 2012, was 2:03:38, set the previous year in Berlin by Patrick Makau, of Kenya. But Mutai was not interested in 2:03:38. Although he made no announcement of his intentions to the media, he wished not only to break Makau's world record, but to annihilate it—to erase those digits from his mind. Neither fame, nor money, was his principal motivation. He needed to run so fast for a simple, private reason: he believed something precious had been stolen from him.

Mutai's grievance dated back eighteen months, to the 2011 Boston Marathon. Mutai had arrived at that race as a serious prospect, with fast second-place finishes at his previous two marathons in Rotterdam and Berlin. At that time, he was, in the sonorous, antiquated parlance of Kenyan marathoners, an athlete who was "picking." To "pick" is to quicken. It can refer equally to a race or a career. *We start slow,* they might say, *and then we* pick.

In Boston, Mutai picked as never before. On the cold morning of April 18, 2011, with a breeze at his back, he beat his countryman Moses Mosop in a thrilling race, and finished in a time of

2:03:02—a course record by nearly three minutes, and almost one minute faster than Haile Gebrselassie's world record of 2:03:59. Mosop finished four seconds behind Mutai, in 2:03:06.

These were absurd, freakish times. Despite its length, the professional marathon is a sport of tiny margins—a few seconds here, a few seconds there. Nobody in the modern era had broken a course record at a major marathon by nearly three minutes before Mutai. Looking on, the American marathon great, Bill Rodgers, who was himself a four-time winner of the Boston Marathon, thought the clocks were broken.

"It was something incredible," said Rodgers. "I ran with a tailwind in Boston one day, and I ran 2:09:55. He ran more than six minutes faster!"

The clocks were working. However, Mutai's run would not stand as an official world record. It is one of many bizarre quirks of the sport of professional road running that, despite being the oldest continuously contested marathon in the world, Boston does not count for world record purposes. Before 2003, when the International Association of Athletics Federations designed regulations so that the marathon could be measured for a world record like any other distance, there had only been marathon "world bests" at 26.2 miles. (The pre-2003 rule was, in many ways, a more satisfactory situation, because it recognized that every marathon course, and every marathon day, is different.) When the IAAF stipulated its criteria, it decreed that a world record must be run on a looped course, with the start and finish separated by no more than 50 percent of the distance, and that the net downhill must be no greater than 1 meter per kilometer. Boston, which runs in a straight shot from Hopkinton, Massachusetts, to the city's downtown, and which is downhill on aggregate, fails to fulfill these conditions.

These thoughts—of the record, and its ineligibility in Boston—had not entered Mutai's mind until the finish line. Boston is not traditionally considered a fast race. It has plenty of hills, and employs no pacemakers. Only a fool would start the Boston Marathon in the hope or expectation of breaking a world record.

During the race itself, Mutai's pacing calculations had been thrown off by his failure to properly analyze the lead vehicle's display—which showed minutes per mile, rather than the kilometers he was accustomed to. Occasionally he would see a metric marker, but the numbers would not compute. (At 30km, he read the split and thought, *Wow! What is this?* He then wondered whether to trust the numbers he had seen.) Of course, he knew within himself that he was running quickly—his body was in a kind of delicious agony—but he had no idea *how* quickly. And so he simply dedicated himself to besting his closest rival and winning the race.

It was only when he crested the line in first place, and hugged his Dutch manager, Gerard Van de Veen, that he began to process what he had just accomplished. He looked at the clock: 2:03:02. A crazy time. And then Van de Veen broke the news that his run in Boston would be only a personal best—that the world record had evaded him because of a technicality. What was worse, everyone started talking about the twenty-mile-an-hour wind that had blown that day. The way people now had it, Mutai had effectively been escorted to the finish line by a hurricane. Not only was his time not an official world record, but it was also adorned with asterisks.

Mutai was wounded. He knew there had been a tailwind in Boston that day. But Boston is hilly. And even downhills, he knew, destroyed the legs. What's more, he thought, where were those asterisks in all those races where a gale blew in his face? And, even more galling, why was he given no credit for the fact that he and Mosop had fought to maintain their speed without the aid of professional pacemakers?

In short, he believed in what he had achieved—wind or no wind, hills or no hills. In the form of his life, driven on by a fierce competitor, he had been possessed by the Spirit, and run an unprecedented time. Those kinds of days didn't come around too often. Marathon running is a tough, capricious sport. Mutai knew he might never rediscover that alchemic combination of shape, conditions, and competition that had pushed him to such an extraordinary performance. And now people wanted to tell him it didn't count?

"It was painful," he said. "It hurt me. But then I sit down and I tell myself, 'This is not the end.' . . ."

Mutai made a pledge. Before he retired, he would beat 2:03:02 on a recognized course in unimpeachable circumstances. Even when his countryman Patrick Makau broke the world record in Berlin, in September 2011, Mutai paid it little mind. He had run faster than Makau's official world record, and would do so again. He believed in his gift. He would silence the talkers. Two-oh-two or die trying. Nothing else could satisfy him.

——

September 29, 2012, was a good day for a man with such intentions. Many factors must align for the marathon world record to fall. One of them is the weather. The conditions should be chilly, dry, near windless—just as it was in Berlin that morning. The spectators wore gloves and sunglasses, and there was only the lightest of southwesterly breezes. On the Strasse des 17. Juni, where Reagan once implored Gorbachev to "tear down this wall," the leaves had turned the color of used teabags, and the Brandenburg Gate framed a cloudless cerulean sky.

Mutai knew that any further incursions into the world record would reignite the long-smoldering debate about the possibility of the first sub-two-hour marathon. The argument about the feasibility of that performance raged both between fans and between scientists, and became increasingly heated whenever the world record fell. But, the way Mutai understood it, the debate was framed front to back. It missed the point.

Mutai had no doubt that running 26 miles and 385 yards in less than two hours was physically possible. The performance, he believed, was within his own body. What stopped marathoners from running faster, he believed, was not so much the structure of their bodies as the structure of races. There was no point thinking about the two-hour marathon when you saw how the sport existed in 2012—namely, a few exceptional athletes lined up twice a year in a great world city, barreling 26.2 miles through the streets. Occasionally, at night in his mountain hideaway, Mutai would fantasize about how the sport might evolve so that it became more about the limits of physiology than about winners and losers. He knew that in the right set of circumstances, people could run so much faster.

These were dreams for another day. Mutai focused on what he could realistically achieve on Berlin's broad, gorgeous avenues. Two-oh-two and change was, he believed, within his compass.

The race directors were naturally keen for Mutai to break the world record. For a niche sport like professional marathon running, record times at a Sunday marathon are sometimes the only way to generate a Monday headline. So, between the organizers, the athletes, and Mutai's manager, a plan was drawn up. The pacemakers were to take the lead pack through the halfway mark in 61 minutes and 30 seconds. If all went according to schedule, Mutai would finish the race in an "even" split (for exactly two hours and three minutes), or he would run the second half faster than the first for a "negative" split of 2:02 and change.

To a marathon runner of almost any standard, these numbers are enough to provoke nightmares. For an elite competitor, one's predicted halfway split time is significant because it is a marker of what one hopes to achieve in the race. The marathon is, at its highest level, a delicate exercise in expending energy evenly over the entire course, and the fastest times are generally achieved when the second half of the race is run at the same speed (an "even" split) as, or slightly faster (a "negative" split) than, the first. Sudden rises or dips in pace can kill a record attempt stone dead. At many marathons, race organizers employ pacemakers, or "rabbits"—other athletes who for reasons of schedule, finance, or talent are paid a few thousand dollars each to run only a limited section of the race—to ensure that the lead athlete's desired pace is adhered to, and to offer some protection against the wind. The rabbits are generally paid by distance: some will travel to halfway, some to 25km, and the strongest to 30km or 32km. From there, the racers are on their own.

At the prerace technical meeting in a drab conference room at Berlin's Maritim Hotel, at noon on the day before the marathon, it was confirmed that Mutai had asked the rabbits to take him through halfway in 61:30. No athlete in the history of the sport had ever asked for such a fast split, but the other Kenyans in the room didn't flinch. At least four of them felt confident that they could run 61:30 for the first half and still finish strong. However, when Jan Fitschen—an affable German marathon runner in the twilight of a career in which he had won, among other honors, the European 10,000m gold medal—was asked about the split Mutai had requested, he made an unfamiliar sound, somewhere between a giggle and a cough. A few minutes later, when the meeting was finished, he walked away shaking his head and laughing. Fitschen hoped to run the first half of the race in 67 minutes.

Ten years earlier, running the first half in 62 minutes and 30 seconds was considered suicidal. When Haile Gebrselassie ran his first marathon in London, in 2002, he asked the pacemakers for this very split—62:30—to widespread amazement. There was a belief that if a runner, even one as talented as Gebrselassie, were to start so fast, he would inevitably "blow up" in the second half of the race as his energy reserves dwindled and lactic acid flooded his muscles. A 62:30 split, it was thought, was a sure and painful way to lose money.

One of Haile's competitors for the 2002 London Marathon was the world record holder Khalid Khannouchi, who was raised in Morocco and became an American citizen in 2000. When Khannouchi's wife, Sandra, heard about the split Haile had proposed, she was apparently so incensed that she made a noisy demonstration of her feelings at the prerace technical meeting. There was no way, she said, that her husband would be joining this idiotic early pace. But come halfway, Khannouchi was with Haile and the other challenger, Paul Tergat—and evidently the pace did not finish him off. He went on to win the race and break the world record in 2:05:38.

Strange things had happened to professional marathon running since 2002. Not only had two minutes fallen from the world record, but the distance appeared to have changed genre. By 2012, the elite no longer considered the marathon a pure endurance event. It was a *speed*-endurance event. The world's best had, in the words of the American commentator Toni Reavis, "outtrained the distance." To explain the difference, many of the most experienced coaches used an automotive analogy. It used to be the case that marathon runners needed a diesel engine. Now the best had turbo-diesels. They were capable of both doughty endurance and devastating pace.

——

Within 5km of the startline in Berlin, a disaster occurred. The display on the pace car froze. The time it showed was 2 minutes and 50 seconds per kilometer. (A marathon run at this pace would finish in 1:59:33.) But the speed the lead group was actually running was around 3 minutes per kilometer, good enough only for a 2:06 finish. For a few klicks, the athletes appeared not to have noticed that they were being fed erroneous information. In fact, Maiyo later said that for the first part of the race, the group actively held the pace back on account of the frozen display, believing they were running too fast. It wasn't ridiculous, he said, to believe that they were traveling at a 2:50/km pace, per se. The whole group had run in the 2:40s per kilometer while running sub-one-hour half marathons.

There is some dispute as to when, exactly, the pacemakers and Mutai's group discovered the mistake. The lead group was accompanied by at least three motorcycles, which carried the race organizer Mark Milde, as well as two athlete managers, both from Holland: Van de Veen of Volare Sports, who represented Mutai and Kimetto, and Valentijn Trouw of Global Sports Communication, who represented Maiyo and Kamworor. Managers are not permitted to coach during the race, but they were within their rights to tell Milde about the frozen screen on the pace car. At least one of the pacemakers was also wearing a GPS watch.

However they were alerted, the athletes in the lead group understood the problem sometime between the fifth and the tenth kilometer, and raised their pace accordingly. But the delay might already have cost them a shot at the world record. The time they lost in the confusion could be recovered later, but maybe at too great a cost. They would need to accelerate sharply, and world record attempts are rarely successful when there is a dramatic spike in pace.

Of course, Mutai would not have been thinking in this way. Marathon runners, by default, must have resilient minds. He set about retrieving his vanished seconds. Having recovered somewhat, he was led along with his competitors through the halfway mark in 1:02:12, some 42 seconds down on his intended split.

By his own recollection, it was only at halfway that he seriously considered the scale of the challenge confronting him. Having run the first half slower than he had hoped, he understood dimly that the sub-2:03 marathon was gone already. But he still believed he had a shot at Makau's world record of 2:03:38. In order to break it, he would need to run the second half of the race in 61:26. Only two men in history had run that fast in the second half of a marathon: the Brazilian athlete Ronaldo da Costa, in Berlin, in 2003, after a sluggish first half; and Mutai himself, on that windy day in Boston, in 2011. The question was: Did Mutai have the legs? Was he the same athlete who had recalibrated the world of marathon running in 2011?

Mutai would not die wondering what might have been. In previous races, he had proved a ferocious competitor. In the next 10km, just as the course rose slightly in gradient, he caught fire. At 25km, as planned, two rabbits dropped out, leaving the lead group paced by only one man—Victor Kipchirchir, a training partner of Mutai's. The pace quickened. Jonathan Maiyo felt tight and began to weaken. He was soon dropped from the lead group. Geoffrey Kamworor also failed to respond to the rising pace in his first marathon and lost touch with the leaders shortly afterward. At 30km, the final rabbit, Kipchirchir, made his scheduled exit.

Now it was only Kimetto and Mutai, head-to-head for the final quarter of the race. As they had done many times together, training at nearly 9,000 feet on the rough hills around their base in the forests of Kenya, they drove each other on. From 30km to 35km, the pair ran a 14:18 split, which is absurdly fast. (A whole marathon run at this pace would finish in 2 hours and 40 seconds.) As Mutai led the charge, with his stiff-backed protégé at his shoulder, he dipped his head in trademark fashion, and a hint of a snarl appeared at the corner of his mouth—a look he refers to as "Now, business."

Within his body, there was a tumult of exertion. His lion's heart pistoned at more than 160 beats per minute. His lungs bellowed half a gallon with every breath. He took three strides a second. In his cells, a complex process was taking place to power his heart and lungs and legs—the burning and resynthesizing of adenosine triphosphate (or ATP)—creating three times as much heat as it did energy. And so he was hot, too hot. His body, losing around three liters of sweat an hour, grew slick with moisture.

Lactic acid began to singe his muscles. Everything but his conscious mind screamed *Stop!* And still he ran.

How does it feel to travel so fast, so late in a marathon? Mutai described the sensation as "fighting inside"—as if your body is at war with itself. Another former runner said it was like putting your hand in a bowl of hot water. You have to keep your hand in, while the water just keeps getting hotter and hotter. Take your hand out, and you lose the race.

Mutai is, of course, accustomed to these sensations. In the four or five months of specific training he undertakes before each major marathon, he runs around 125 miles a week. His total mileage in that period is the equivalent of running in a straight line from New York City to Los Angeles. Moreover, the training is savage—up and down hills, at altitude, at alternating speeds, on rough roads. Many sessions, he says, are much harder than a race. Indeed, while competing, the natural discomfort of powering his body along at 13 miles an hour is balanced by the joy he feels in doing it. If training has allowed Mutai to breathe the Spirit, a race should feel like one steady exhalation.

However good his preparation has been, there are moments in races when Mutai needs to fetch water from a deep well. After halfway in Berlin, he lowered the rope, hand over hand. Mutai recalls, in this moment of profound athletic endeavor, that he drew strength from the crowds that lined the roads. He said he could feel that "people love me" and he determined to repay that affection with a Herculean effort—to consciously override the signals his body was sending him. "I sacrificed myself," he remembered.

At 35km, the sacrifice appeared to have paid off. Despite the botched beginning, both Mutai and Kimetto were now inside world record pace. All they had to do was hold on. If they ran a 2:56/km pace for the final 7.2km of the race—which seemed, given their earlier pace, to be possible—the world record would fall to one or the other.

Perhaps inevitably, they couldn't do it. The prodigious acceleration just after halfway exacted its reward, and, by 40km, slowing markedly, both athletes were eight seconds outside world record pace and spent. Mutai's right hamstring began to tighten—the product, he believed, of slipping on wet mud while completing his training in unseasonably rainy conditions at home. The pain moved to his hip and back. He wanted desperately to stop. He believed that if he had done so, even for a second, his race would have been over. He couldn't look left or right. His pain was so great that he said he could not bend to take a water bottle at 40km. And still, Kimetto—high-shouldered, and seemingly in better shape—ran at his back.

Facing the final two kilometers, this unhappy pair ran into the breeze, rather slowly. They seemed headed for a very fast time, but not a world record. For the crowd on the home straightaway, there was at least the prospect of a manful tussle to see which athlete would prevail. And, as Mutai and Kimetto ran through the Brandenburg Gate shoulder to shoulder, 400 meters from the end, the spectators raised their voices in anticipation of a sprint finish.

But the kick never came. In a finale in which a burst from either man would have sealed the race decisively, Kimetto finished the race as he had run most of it: just behind his colleague. Mutai raised his arms weakly as he crested the line in a time of 2:04:15. It was the celebration of a boxer whose opponent could not lift himself from his stool, not the roar of a fighter who had knocked out an adversary. Seconds later, the two men shared a limp, exhausted hug.

Why no sprint? There were half a million reasons why. If Kimetto had beaten his training partner, Mutai might have lost the $500,000 World Marathon Majors jackpot—money that Kimetto had no chance of winning himself, this being his first marathon. Meanwhile, Kimetto was not just Mutai's training partner. For the previous few years, like many in the village where he trained, he had been fed and housed by Mutai. If he had sprinted past his boss under the Brandenburg Gate, everyone in that village would have lost. When Mutai won, everyone in the village—and many others—won. Marathon runners are not just athletes; they are economies.

The tacit arrangement between the two men seemed obvious to most observers with some knowledge of the sport. But when Van de Veen was later confronted about the apparent pact, he was furious. "There was no deal!" he told journalists.

As a statement of literal fact, Van de Veen might be correct—there may have been no exchange of words between his two athletes. There wouldn't have to be. Kimetto is a quiet man, but he is not stupid. For his part, Mutai said both he and Kimetto were dog tired at the close of the race and neither man could have done anything more. Of course, Mutai may be right. And, of course, he would say that. We will never know.

Mutai's finishing time of 2:04:15 was the fastest time that anybody ran in 2012. For the second year in a row, he was the quickest marathoner on the planet. But these statistics brought him little comfort. Although, in the aftermath of the race, he signed autographs and smiled for photographs, he left Berlin with the sense of an opportunity lost—of a tide untaken.

Chapter Two

The Dreamers Among Us

T HE WAY Mike Joyner remembers it, the dream of the two-hour marathon began its life as a hangover in Tucson, Arizona, in December 1977. Joyner was a nineteen-year-old undergraduate at the University of Arizona: tall, skinny, smart as hell, and utterly uninterested in an academic career. He recalls his priorities at the time were running track, chasing girls, and drinking beer—not necessarily in that order. He had decided to drop out of college and take the test to become a Tucson city firefighter.

One night before running a 10km race at the San Xavier del Bac Catholic mission, just south of Tucson, Joyner had "a little too much fun." He showed up for the race hungover, and ran with all the energy of a tequila worm. In the last mile or so, he was caught by a graduate student from the university named Eddie Coyle—a good miler, but a guy Joyner should have beaten easily, had his preparations been more abstemious.

After the race, the two men started chatting. Coyle was working on exercise physiology for his doctorate, under a pioneering scientist named Jack Wilmore, and was trying to recruit human guinea pigs for a study about "lactate threshold" in runners. Joyner said he'd do it. Days later, Coyle hooked Joyner up to a few machines as he ran on a treadmill.

Joyner was intrigued by the experiment—about the process, and about what the process was attempting to test. He forgot about being a firefighter and stayed in college. His grades improved. He started to focus on science. He contributed to Wilmore's graduate journal club as an undergraduate and worked as a lab technician on his vacations. His path was set: he wanted to know the secrets of an athlete's body. The question was, how to do it? Joyner noticed that much of the best work in the field of exercise physiology was being done by Scandinavian doctors. He couldn't do much about being Scandinavian, but he could become a medical doctor. He decided to study for his MD.

Joyner's curiosity was—and remains—insatiable. As a medical student, he became fascinated by the thresholds of sporting endeavor, and in particular, the idea of a runner's limits. In 1986, before he'd graduated from medical school, Joyner began thinking about the two-hour marathon. He'd been working on papers that investigated how measures like lactate threshold, running economy, and VO_2 max (or lung capacity)—all of which have a limiting effect on running speed and endurance—related to athletic performance. What would it be possible for a human being to run, he wondered, if he had the *best possible* values for lactate threshold, running economy, and VO_2 max? He drew up a model and came to a surprisingly specific number. Given ideal conditions, and the ideal runner, Joyner concluded that the best time in which a marathon could be completed was 1 hour, 57 minutes, and 58 seconds.

He wrote up his findings and tried to find a publisher. It took him five years, but eventually his paper—peer-reviewed, and rubber-stamped—appeared in the *Journal of Applied Physiology* in 1991. It became the seminal document in the two-hour-marathon debate and catalyzed a fierce argument in the scientific and running community that continues to this day. Joyner is now a professor of anesthesiology, and has been working with distinction at the Mayo Clinic in Rochester, Minnesota, since 1987, on a wide range of topics—from gene studies to cardiovascular disease—but none has stuck to him as much as his famous 1991 paper. He gets asked more questions about his undergraduate work on the two-hour marathon than about anything else.

1:57:58. The implications of that number were obvious to anybody with even a passing interest in distance running. It meant the two-hour marathon was attainable—in theory, at least. At the time of the study's publication, the world's fastest marathon was 2:06:50, and the two-hour mark existed only at the far reaches of the imagination: the Narnia of distance running. Joyner was the first person to apply some scientific rigor to the question of whether two hours was actually possible. And, according to him, it was.

———

The two-hour debate is irresistible, inevitable. It arises every time a man breaks the marathon world record. In 2003, for instance, Paul Tergat crested the tape at the Berlin Marathon in 2:04:55. Before that race, only "world bests" were recognized. Tergat's time, which crushed Khalid Khannouchi's seventeen-month-old world best by 43 seconds, was the first ratified marathon "world record."

At the postrace press conference in Berlin, the victor was asked *the* question. "I believe records are set to be broken, and to fall lower is possible," said Tergat. "But what remains impossible is running a marathon in under two hours." He then smiled, and added: "Maybe time will chide me."

Time has a chiding habit. The history of athletics is also the history of bad predictions. Take the case of the Australian John Landy, one of the world's best middle-distance runners in the early 1950s. At the peak of his powers, he yearned to become the first man to break four minutes for the mile, and many believed he had the heart and the talent to do so. But, after several tilts at the barrier, in which he failed by two or three seconds each time, he declared himself defeated.

"It is a brick wall," said Landy in April 1954. "I shall not attempt it again."

It was not a brick wall. On May 6, 1954, despite dire prognostications from armchair pundits, some of whom believed a human would die if he attempted to run a mile in under four minutes, a junior doctor named Roger Bannister ran 3:59.4 for the mile at the Iffley Road running track in Oxford, England.

The world of athletics moved on fast. Six weeks after Bannister made history, Landy himself obliterated the new world record, running 3:58 dead. In the years that followed, sub-four-minute miles became commonplace among elite athletes. (In 2011, the fifth American high school boy broke the barrier.) The four-minute mile was only unbreakable until one man broke it. "Après moi," said Bannister, "le déluge."

Within the next few years—or decades, depending on whom you listen to—another brick wall will crumble when a marathon is run in less than two hours. Before that moment, there will continue to be well-placed onlookers who think a sub-two marathon will never be run. Their opinions will stem from strong roots. When Tergat told the press conference it "remains impossible" to run a marathon in under two hours, he was reflecting on the abyss into which he had just pushed his own body in order to run 2:04:55. In that moment, the prospect of running a whole five minutes faster than his new world record was unfathomable.

Five minutes in a marathon is too much slack for the brain to handle. But nobody is suggesting a 1:59:59 marathon will be reached in one giant leap. In 2011, a new world record of 2:03:38 was set by Patrick Makau, in Berlin. That performance beat Haile Gebrselassie's 2:03:59 from 2008 by 21 seconds, which in turn beat Gebrselassie's previous best from 2007 by 27 seconds, which beat Tergat's landmark of 2:04:55.

Tim Noakes, one of the world's leading exercise physiologists, and the author of the influential book *Lore of Running*, believes that these incremental advances are connected to how the brains of top athletes communicate with their bodies.

"When you start running," he says, "you know what the world record is, so you don't have to run ten minutes faster than the world record. Your whole focus is to run one second faster than the world record. That's what your brain is keyed in on. And that programming occurs all the time in running and is terribly important."

The brains of elite athletes are only as obstructive as they are programmed to be—as one recent, brilliant experiment showed. In 2011, at around the same time that Geoffrey Mutai was tearing up the marathon world, Professor Kevin Thompson of the University of Northumbria, in northeast England, assembled a group of enthusiastic bike riders for a laboratory test. These cyclists were placed on stationary bikes in front of screens, hooked up to oxygen monitors, and asked to race a computer-generated cyclist avatar. Each rider had previously set a personal best for a 4,000m time trial on the machine. The avatar they were now racing represented that personal best.

Or so these guinea pig cyclists thought. In fact, Thompson was lying. He had set the avatar to race 2 percent faster than their personal bests because he wanted to know if an athlete's body could be tricked into performing better. It was his belief that even world-class performers, who thought they were regulating their energy output to their absolute maximum, possessed a "reserve" of around 2 percent that could be tapped into, given the right motivation (or a little deception).

Thompson was right. Almost all of the cyclists finished ahead of the avatar. When they were told about the stunt that Thompson and his colleagues had pulled, a few aired their suspicions about how tough the ride had been compared to their earlier attempts. But the fact remained: the mind could be tricked. All the cyclists believed that when they set their personal bests they were cycling as hard as they could. They weren't. Bodies have more than one limit. An athlete's brain, constantly walking the tightrope between regulating exhaustion and maximizing performance, plays games to stay alive. So, why break the world record by two minutes when you can break it by two seconds?

—

If two hours is reached, it will be in such baby steps—each one taken by a member of the tiny, elite fraternity of athletes with the talent and industry to inch the sport closer to the impossible marathon, world record by world record. In Berlin, Geoffrey Mutai was only the latest in a more than century-long line of pioneers who had engaged in this multigenerational quest.

The pioneer will also have been the beneficiary of intellectual progress. Records fall because of technical innovation as much as physiological improvement. The Fosbury Flop revolutionized the high jump; the somersault turn shaved seconds off swimming records. Running may seem to be the most rudimentary of sports, but there are countless ways in which the runners of today are blessed with advantages their predecessors were not: better shoes, better training ideas, better racing conditions.

To the freethinker, there are still gains to be made in all these areas. Take the road itself. The Olympic champion Seb Coe believes the cinder track on which Roger Bannister set his first sub-four-minute mile sixty years ago is one and a half seconds a lap slower than the tracks of today. Meanwhile, it is beyond doubt that the current generation of marathon runners is not racing on the most conducive surface.

In 1977, Peter Greene and Tom McMahon built something they called a "tuned track" at Harvard University. It improved runners' times by nearly 3 percent. The construction of the tuned track stemmed from a particular interest that the two men shared—that of matching the springlike qualities of tendons and muscles to an ideal running surface. They believed, correctly, that too hard a track was sapping for a distance runner, and too soft a track drained energy from their legs. The perfect springiness would reside somewhere between these two points, and might vary from runner to runner. Having found a rough sweet spot, they made their track at Harvard using wood, topped by polyurethane. And everyone, without fail, ran faster.

If you wanted to create a miles-long, all-weather version of

Greene and McMahon's surface, perfectly tuned for marathon-ers, you'd encounter several obstacles, not least the cost. Perhaps the biggest problem is that the IAAF rules state that a marathon must be run on "made-up road," by which they mean the regular tarmac you see on city streets, and so any record set on a track would be unofficial. But if you really wanted to see what was possible in the marathon, you'd find a way to move the world's best runners off the asphalt.

——

As Tergat recognized, it is in the nature of humans to progress. In the first Olympic marathon, in 1896, only the Greek winner, Spyridon Louis, broke three hours. Now any club runner worth his salt can run faster. In 119 years since that catalyzing race, the world record has reflected prodigious improvements in life-style, technology, training methods, and psychology, as athletes have brought down the time in fits and starts. Two-oh-three and change would have been a science-fiction performance to Spyridon Louis, but it exists today. The impossible becomes possible. Time chides.

Besides, champions are in an uncomfortable position to make accurate predictions because they necessarily see the sport through the prism of their own superlative achievements. Bill Rodgers, who won four Boston Marathons and four New York City Marathons between 1976 and 1980, was interviewed by *Track & Field News* in 1977, at a time when the fastest marathon ever run had been recorded by an Australian, Derek Clayton—a 2:08:33 he ran on a disputed course in Antwerp, Belgium, in 1969. Nobody, including Rodgers, had come close to running so fast since, and the American was asked by the interviewer whether he believed the marathon world record had reached a plateau. "It seems so," said Rodgers.

Clayton himself was only marginally less pessimistic. In his career, during which he held down a job as a draftsman while clocking 200-mile training weeks, he became the first man to break 2:10 for the marathon. His world best of 2:08:33, meanwhile, was not broken for twelve years. In 1980, he wrote a short and somewhat lifeless book called *Running to the Top* that was remarkable only for this statement: "For the rest of my life I will watch with interest to see how my 2:08:33 stands the test of time. I might live long enough to see a 2:06 [but] a two hour marathon—4.34 mile pace—definitely not."

Clayton may be right about not seeing a sub-two-hour marathon in his lifetime. But he is still very much alive and well and living in Melbourne, Australia, and the world best is three minutes better than he predicted. Rodgers's "plateau" has proven to be further off. These men are not foolish. They understand their sport intimately. But when it comes to making predictions in athletics, time, as Tergat noted, runs a canny race.

It's not just athletes who make poor predictions. Scientists and physiologists are notoriously lousy at seeing around corners. Edward "Ned" Frederick, who worked for many years at the Nike Sport Research Lab, wrote a fascinating paper in 1986 in which he charted the history of pessimism in the performance prediction business. In 1906, for instance, Harvard's Arthur Kennelly calculated the best time in which it was possible for a human to run a mile. Kennelly's ultimate mile was 3 minutes and 58.7 seconds.

At the time the Harvard scientist made his prediction, the world's best time for the mile was 4:15.6. It would take nearly fifty years for Kennelly to be proved wrong. In fact, it was John Landy, the same runner who claimed that four minutes for the mile was a brick wall, who eventually bettered Kennelly's "best possible" time in June 1954, with his 3:58-dead in Turku, Finland. But the world record is now way beyond Kennelly's imagining. It stands at 3:43.13, set in 1999 by the Moroccan Hicham El Guerrouj— some 15 seconds faster than Kennelly deemed possible.

Frederick's lesson from these well-meaning bungles is simple. When it comes to sports, the future is a foreign country. He wrote:

> Ever since such records have been kept they have been inexorably broken, much to the puzzlement of scientists . . . who delight in this ancient, armchair sport of calculating the ultimate. What keeps these predictors continually sharpening their pencils and redefining the limits is the simple idea that there must be intrinsic limits to how high, how far, and how fast the fittest of our species can propel themselves. After all, no reasonable person would think that a human will someday run the mile in 5.4 microseconds (i.e., at the speed of light) or high jump over the moon, and few would disagree that the current records will be broken. Our scientific guesswork focuses on the vast territory in between. It is tempting to assume that there is an ultimate, a limit to human performance which we can predict, but this may not be the case.

—— ——

Why does it matter whether the sub-two-hour marathon is possible? And if it is possible, what will it mean when the first 1:59:59 marathon is run? At one level, the achievement will signify nothing. To complete 26 miles and 385 yards in less than two hours using only one's God-given gifts would be, of course, an exceptional feat of speed, mental strength, and endurance. But the marathon length is a scruffy figure, only fixed by the Olympic Committee in 1921 to match the course of the 1908 London Olympic marathon, which was itself designed to accommodate the peculiar viewing demands of the British royal family. Why should we care if some extraordinary person can run this arbitrary distance in just over, or just under, two hours?

For curious reasons, we do care and it does matter. Twenty-six miles and 385 yards is not just a distance. It has become a metaphor. Nobody finds the marathon easy—even professionals, especially professionals. The distance is democratic that way. Everyone who runs a marathon is running against his or her limits. Everyone is forced to manage a certain amount of pain and to recruit hidden reserves. Whatever one's talent or preparation, nobody runs an easy marathon. Geoffrey Mutai's prayer at the startline is not to win the race, but to finish it.

On the other side of the coin, the marathon is also a race that is possible for almost anyone with enough patience and willpower to complete. The distance is democratic that way, too. For this reason, it has become an event against which hordes of every-day people—fat people, thin people; people crooked by time and people sprightly as foals; rich people and people in need—test themselves. I'm running against cancer. I'm running for my dad. I'm running for a personal best. As Chris Brasher, cofounder of the London Marathon, once said, the race has become "the great suburban Everest."

Now, in the popular imagination, the marathon is not primarily a test of athletic talent, but a test of character. The race has become a carnival of men and women, some in outrageous costumes, each attempting to overcome a personal hurdle for the public good, or a public hurdle for a personal good. A British man named Lloyd Scott is perhaps the most extreme of these charitable masochists. Among other stunts, he has completed both the New York and London marathons in an antiquated deep-sea diving suit weighing 130 pounds, and has raised nearly £5 million for charity in the past decade. When he received the MBE (Member of the British Empire) honor from the Queen for his fund-raising feats, he said that it should stand for "Mad, Bonkers, and Eccentric."

The madness is spreading. There are now more than five hundred marathons all over the world, and more entrants into races than at any time in the history of the sport. But as the marathon has blossomed as a general participation event, it has for many ceased to hold interest as an elite contest. The event is now utterly dominated by East Africans, and there is only one widely recognized elite marathon runner—Haile Gebrselassie, whose glory days are long behind him. Even committed runners can be indifferent to the achievements of the best in their sport. If one were to ask every single finisher of the New York City Marathon who held the world record at the distance they had just completed, the majority would not know.

Unless you are one of the minority of sports fans interested in elite distance running—and it is a tiny cadre of obsessives—a glance at the startline of a major marathon yields not a single familiar face. What you see is a parade of gaunt, lithe black men with low numbers on their vests, arrayed in the lurid uniforms of shoe companies. Their names are as good as indistinguishable, and their stories mysterious.

The only thing you would understand about these men is that they are fast. You know that their pale-skinned competitors—Europeans and Japanese and American elite runners, who seem equally gaunt and lithe—have no chance to win the race. East Africans win marathons; Kenyans, particularly. Pluck one dreamy statistic from the pack: in 2011, all five World Marathon Majors (in Boston, London, Berlin, Chicago, and New York) were won by Kenyans. All were run in a new course record.

But what do we really know of these exceptional men, except their trade? We know nothing of their homes, or families, or desires, or vices. We do not know if one of them drinks too much, or beats his wife. We do not know which one has dreamed of the moment we are now witnessing all of his life, through years of honest toil, and whose stomach is now knotted at the prospect. We do not know how much they are paid. We do not know if one of them cheats.

We do not know any of this because their gut-wrenching labors, both during the race and in the months preceding it, are painted effortless: a beautiful trick. Meanwhile, at the finishing line, the chances are the victor will react the same, whoever he is. Confronted by a white man with a microphone and a television camera, he will give thanks to God in a voice so gentle it would not snuff a candle placed by his mouth, thank the organizers of the race, and then return home to spend his winnings.

All of this is disguise. The professional marathon is a savage, enthralling sport, and not only because of the demands it places on the body. Many of its greatest protagonists—who seem possessed of an enviable lightness—carry with them the heavy reckoning of wretched childhoods. It is no exaggeration to say that the man who runs the first sub-two-hour marathon will have overcome not only a sporting challenge but an existential one.

Haile Gebrselassie once asked me, "You think you can be a successful runner from a good family?" It was not really a question. He had talked of his upbringing in Ethiopia: about the poverty that surrounded him, and about the violence meted out to him in his home. Haile's counterintuitive analysis was that all world-beating runners spring from twisted roots. He believed that a deficit of opportunities, and an early taste of pain, had not stifled his talent but fertilized it.

——

Haile's insight into the genesis of his own greatness holds a clue not only to the emotional conformation of the athletes who drive the sport onward but also to the appeal of the distance. The marathon is a race that tethers runners to their own personal narratives. It is, as Gebrselassie says, "a question of how you grow." On race day—with the barest equipment, no teammates, and scant protection from the elements—you are as good as naked. Nothing but your own body will sustain you; everything you have done in your life until the moment you cross the finishing line is connected to the effort.

But the lure of the marathon goes beyond this. There are those who argue that long footraces are at the heart of our evolution as a species. In 2004, a now-famous paper written by two evolutionary anthropologists, Dennis Bramble and Dan Lieberman, was published on the cover of *Nature* magazine, and titled "Endurance Running and the Evolution of *Homo*." Its central contention was revolutionary: human beings evolved as they did because they were expert at endurance hunting—running down their prey over many miles.

"From head to toe, it just works," they argued. "We evolved to run."

This portrait—known as the Running Man theory—has been given plenty of oxygen, most notably in Christopher McDougall's popular book *Born to Run*. It is worth reprising the key points. In the Running Man theory, several evolutionary markers seem to point to our development as endurance hunters. For instance, unlike nonrunning mammals, but like horses and dogs, we can hold our heads still at high speeds because of the nuchal ligament at the base of our skulls. We also have strong gluteus muscles to power our legs and to counterbalance our heavy chests. Our feet and ankles are spring-loaded with tendons and ligaments that we need to run. We have narrow waists that allow us to swing our arms and legs in a straight line. Most important, we sweat. Because our bodies cool themselves, we can outrun a furry quadruped and have him for dinner.

A South African scientist named Louis Liebenberg spent years observing Kalahari bushmen—some of the last endurance hunters on earth—as they ran down antelope over long distances, in searing midday heat. These hunts took up to six or eight hours, but the humans generally prevailed. Liebenberg noted how, in the final few kilometers, the hunters he observed entered "a trancelike state." Eventually, in the successful pursuits, the animal collapsed, exhausted. The only weapons the bushmen needed were their minds and their bodies. Liebenberg is convinced that endurance hunting holds the key to our development as a species.

The Running Man theory posits that endurance hunting was crucial to early humans because of our lust for protein. In order to feed our growing brains, we needed meat. Without the sprint speed to surprise animals on the savannah, we developed another strategy: run them to death. One of the most interesting offshoots of the Running Man theory is what it says about our brains. In order to slog five or six hours across the sun-bleached savannah in pursuit of prey in possession of explosive speed, you need to have great powers of imagination—and a capacity to delay gratification.

In his odd and intriguing book *Why We Run,* the biologist Bernd Heinrich explained this "visionary power" that runners must possess. "The key to endurance, as all distance runners know, is not just a matter of sweat glands. It's vision. To endure is to have a clear goal and the ability to extrapolate to it with the mind—the ability to keep in mind what is not before the eye. Vision allows us to reach into the future, whether it's to kill an antelope or to achieve a record time in a race."

Not everyone buys the Running Man theory. The skeptics argue that all of the attributes associated with running by proponents of the theory could also have been associated with walking. They also argue that, at the time in question, Africa would have been too lush to run across in the manner described by the theorists. And, of course, evolution is a complex process. Who can say which need triggered what change? But this much seems clear: however important distance running was to the evolution of *Homo sapiens,* modern marathon runners are reenacting an ancient rite.

More than that. Having watched the world's best modern runners compete, and seen seemingly strong athletes founder,

Heinrich's observation rings true to me: it is heightened vision that separates the champions from the also-rans. Naturally, every man has his physical threshold. An NFL linebacker would struggle to finish a marathon in less than three hours, no matter what his willpower or training are like. But among the most talented athletes, from the most fecund pastures of distance running, it is the ability to plan a race, to respond to unexpected difficulties, to hold many possibilities in one's head, and to outwit opponents, that distinguishes a champion. This is true both of an athlete's performance in a race and, perhaps more significant, of his ability to prepare himself for that performance.

The best marathon races, then, are tests not only of conditioning but of intelligence and temperament. Although the sport's leading proponents mostly hail from the same spot on the planet, they are—as a group of American, Japanese, or Icelandic people would be—individuals, forged by their particular histories and distinguished not just by talent but by the force of their will. Major marathons are also special because they are scarce. Unlike in most sports, in which athletes play dozens of games in a single season, the best runners compete twice a year at 26.2 miles. Very few marathoners survive for more than a handful of years at the pinnacle of their sport. They know they have only a few, rare days on which to prove themselves.

The marathon event has undergone a revolution in the past few years, and the world's best male runners can see, but not touch, the near-mythic two-hour mark. Hearing the cream of the current generation discuss the sub-two-hour marathon—half pushing away the very notion of its possibility, and half embracing it as within their compass—there are echoes of the British mountaineer George Mallory, who was the first man to lead a serious assault on Mount Everest. Mallory led expeditions to Everest in 1921, 1922, and finally in 1924, in the attempt that claimed his life. On the first sortie, in 1921, his party had no clear idea where they were going. There was no map; they drew it by hand as they walked to the foot of the mountain. This, in allegorical terms, is where the world's best runners are today.

Mallory was not only a brave and skilled mountaineer, but a fine writer. Having seen horrors as a soldier in the First World War, his accounts of climbing are laced with the romantic overtones of a man newly liberated from a nightmare. Nowhere is this worldview more pronounced than in his description of Everest, the "great white fang, excrescent from the jaw of the world."

In 1921, Mallory wrote this, of his first experience of glimpsing the summit:

> Mountain shapes are often fantastic seen through a mist. These were like the wildest creation of a dream. A preposterous triangular lump rose out of the depths; its edge came leaping up at an angle of about 70 degrees and ended nowhere. To its left a black serrated crest was hanging in the sky incredibly. Gradually, very gradually, we saw the great mountainsides and glaciers and arêtes, now one fragment now another through the floating rifts, until far higher in the sky than imagination had dared to suggest the white summit of Everest appeared. And in this series of partial glimpses we had seen a whole; we were able to piece together the fragments, interpret the dream.

The average East African runner would never frame the quest for the two-hour marathon in these terms. Unlike Mallory, none has the benefit of an education from Cambridge University. But I have never read a better description of what remains, for the best marathoners, a prize glimpsed in snatches. The two-hour marathon exists somewhere beyond the boundaries of their normal, professional existence. There is a dreamlike, intangible quality to the vision, laced with the prospect of real pain. To reach the summit, the pioneer knows that he must endure more, live braver, plan better, and be luckier than his forebears—and that all of these qualities will likely be insufficient. They know the honor may fall to another generation.

———

Patrick Makau's world record, which Mutai tried and failed to obliterate in Berlin, was still 3 minutes and 38 seconds away from the two-hour mark. What's 218 seconds? It's a pop song; a long commercial break; the time it takes to soft-boil a small egg. In marathon terms, however, those 218 seconds are a lifetime.

To run 2:03:38, one's average pace needs to be a shade over 4 minutes and 42 seconds a mile, or, as the metrically minded Kenyans would think about it, 2 minutes and 55 seconds per kilometer. A marathon run in two hours dead requires an average of 4:35 per mile, or 2:50 per kilometer. It's nearly a 3 percent improvement. In the abstract, this difference seems trifling. In reality, the distance between a 2:03:38 performance and a marathon run 218 seconds quicker is like the distance right now between the best African runners and the best Europeans—which is to say, it's chasmic.

The strangest thing about the two-hour debate is that the closer the world record comes to the landmark, the more the pessimists hold sway. Chief among the naysayers are experts like Ross Tucker, a sports scientist from the University of Cape Town, in South Africa, who hosts an influential blog on endurance sports named sportsscientists.com. He is pessimistic of ever seeing a sub-two-hour marathon in his lifetime—and he's a young man. His reasons are complex but boil down to what he believes is the central truth about elite marathon running in the second decade of the twenty-first century: that the art of pacing has already been refined almost to the point of perfection.

At the time of publication, only four men—Wilson Kipsang, Dennis Kimetto, Emmanuel Mutai (no relation to Geoffrey), and Patrick Makau—had run back-to-back sub-62-minute halves over the course of a marathon. (Geoffrey Mutai and Moses Mosop also ran twin sub-62s in Boston, but their run did not count for world record purposes, for reasons explained in the previous chapter.) Most others who have attempted such a strategy have failed dramatically. Given this record, the idea of someone running back-to-back *one-hour* half marathons seems ludicrous to Tucker. In short, he believes that the current elite are already producing outstanding performances that are near the limit of human possibility. They may be able to shave seconds off the world record. But minutes? That will be the work of generations.

Mike Joyner is more hopeful. He notes that since the 1950s, when year-round training became the norm for the world's best athletes, the marathon world record has decreased by more than 16 minutes. Since the 1960s, when the Africans began competing in athletics, the record has fallen between 1 and 5 minutes per decade. Since the 1980s, the progress has been slower. Depending on where one begins counting, and therefore how quickly one believes marathon times will plateau, the first sub-two marathon will either be run around 2022 (if one begins from the 1960s) or around 2035 (if one begins from the 1980s).

Joyner, then, has no doubt that the two-hour marathon will fall, eventually. During our discussions in 2012 and 2013, he argued that Makau's marathon world record of 2:03:38 was a little "soft." In fact, he believed Geoffrey Mutai's unofficial world best of 2:03:02 was also surpassable in the near future. Historically, there is a statistical correlation between the 10,000m world record and the marathon world record. At various times in history, if one took the 10,000m world record and multiplied it by 4.6 or 4.7, one arrived at the marathon world record. Now, if one multiplies the 10,000m world record (of 26:17.53, held by Kenenisa Bekele of Ethiopia) by 4.7 one arrives pretty much at Makau's 2:03:38. But if one looked at the lower end of the statistical set, and multiplied it by 4.6, one reaches a time of around 2 hours and 1 minute for the marathon. This is a time Joyner believes we're heading for soon.

Joyner's optimism is shared by many in the field. In a paper published in 2012, a statistician and marathon historian named David Martin worked with the researcher Holly Ortlund to predict that the first 1:59:59 marathon would be run between 2029 and 2032.

But even this is not a bold enough prediction for some. Doug Casa, an American sports scientist, believes two hours will fall within a decade. His calculation rests on developments in training and athlete management, advances in shoe and drink technology, and the kind of kinetic momentum that comes when records arrive close enough to a landmark like the two-hour marathon, and the drumbeat starts. But the font of his analysis is an optimism in the capacity of human beings to improve. "We're naïve to think that somehow we're as smart as we can be right now," he told me. "Look at the literature from the 1920s, the 1940s, the 1960s, the 1980s. All those times, people were pretty much saying we were reaching our physiological limits. And each time, they were wrong."

Casa's position is much like Ned Frederick's, and its humility is attractive. We are always tempted to view our own era as the ultimate. How many times have we heard that the current generation of athletes trains as hard at it is possible to train, in the best conditions possible, and that preparation for sporting endeavors cannot improve? In his paper written a quarter of a century ago, Frederick's wisdom was to see this presentism for what it was: bunk. Nineteen eighty-six was the future once, too.

The sub-two-hour marathon may be possible or impossible. Nobody knows for sure—and anybody who says he is certain is either a brave man or a fool. The feat appears to be within the range of human possibility, in terms of physiology, according to the models that exist today. But understanding physiology is only one aspect of understanding running. Human beings are more than hearts and lungs and legs, and the quest for virgin territory more than a battle of swift feet.

——

That's one of the reasons we keep watching. As Frederick wrote in his 1986 paper, "The ultimate limits are beyond the ken of all but the dreamers among us." Fortunately, these dreamers exist. You find them in unlikely places: Rochester, Minnesota; Nijmegen, Holland; Eldoret, Kenya. In the summer of 2011, a Scottish product creator at Adidas named Andy Barr, based in the company's headquarters in Herzogenaurach, Germany, stood up at a staff meeting and said something so provocative it is still discussed among his colleagues today. The company was beginning to think about its product line for elite athletes for the 2013 season, and Barr would be instrumental in the design process. He had created the shoe that Haile Gebrselassie wore to break the world record in 2008, and he had also been a principal in the creation of the shoe that Patrick Makau wore in 2011 when he bettered Haile's record by 21 seconds. And so the young Scotsman stood up in that meeting and said that the company's lodestar should be the idea of a sub-two-hour marathon. Adidas's unofficial "Sub-2" project was born.

Barr is a marathon fan as well as a designer of marathon wear, and he had watched in awe as a string of Kenyans—most of them Adidas athletes—had rewritten the possibilities of running 26.2 miles in the 2011 spring marathon season. Geoffrey Mutai's 2:03:02 in Boston, in particular, sparked his interest. "Everybody said the sub-four mile wasn't possible," Barr explained. "And for a long time, it wasn't possible. All of a sudden, 1954, Bannister breaks four minutes. And then everybody breaks it."

Barr and his fellow designers at Adidas were anxious that they not be misunderstood. The project was very much "unofficial"; it was "a metaphor"; under no circumstances would they want to be openly leading a sub-two charge against their main competitor, Nike. But it was clear that there would be a vast and unquantifiable reward for the shoe company whose athlete broke the barrier. Every world record by an Adidas athlete was a chance to sell more shoes, and making history with the first sub-two marathon would be an unparalleled marketing opportunity. Adidas was not the only company thinking along these lines. Late in 2013, it become public knowledge that Nike was working on its own "sub-two" shoe.

The enthusiasm of multinational sporting apparel companies proves nothing about the feasibility of a 1:59:59 marathon. But it does suggest this: regardless of the pessimism of well-informed dissenters, the two-hour quest will not go away in the popular imagination. It is the sport's Everest. As a species, we are interested in outlandish feats, and our brains cleave to landmarks.

Wherever you stand on the two-hour argument—whether you believe the whole debate is silly and premature, or whether you are sure of witnessing this moment of athletic history in the near future—there are three minutes to be extracted from the marathon world record before two hours is reached. You can be certain that those seconds will not fall easily. But somewhere, in the thin air, there is a runner alive right now who glimpsed a prodigious white fang, excrescent from the jaw of the world, and who will set his mind upon its conquest.

Chapter Three

Welcome to Skyland

January 2008, before and after

T HE HOUSES were on fire in the town of Timboroa. Two thousand eight was only a few days old, and Geoffrey Mutai's new
life had barely begun. At age twenty-six, he had just signed his
first contract with a manager and was deep in training for his
first professional marathon *outside*. *Outside* was anywhere out
of Africa. *Outside* was where you got your shot and made your
money. He had battled for years for this moment. Tens of thousands of hours of training and uncountable heartache had been
expended in its pursuit. Now here he was, two months from his
debut at the Monaco Marathon, in a town called Timboroa, and
the houses were on fire.

The whole country was ripping itself apart in the wake of
a disputed general election, but the violence in the Rift Valley
Province, the heartland of Kenya's running community, was par-

ticularly intense. Here, Kikuyus, whose political champion Mwai Kibaki, the incumbent president, had refused to budge from power, fought battles against the Kalenjins, whose preferred choice had been snubbed in what they believed to be a rigged vote. Timboroa was at the fault line of the crisis.

Mutai arrived that day by bicycle. He was still an unknown athlete, but he'd recently won a local race in which the bike was first prize. Now, instead of walking the twenty-five miles or so from his home village of Equator, where his grandparents lived, to his training base in the hills, he could cycle. Mutai was pedaling back to Equator when he passed through Timboroa.

He saw groups of Kikuyu men armed with *pangas*— machetes—moving from building to building. They were hunting Kalenjins: Geoffrey's people. There was no way Mutai could turn around and go back. He had been spotted. He decided to approach the vigilantes. He was terrified. He thought he was going to die.

Although Mutai was unarmed, he possessed two weapons, both of which he deployed in this moment of peril. He spoke fluent Kikuyu, a product of spending several years in a school some distance south, in Rongai, with predominantly Kikuyu classmates. And, despite being in his mid-twenties, he had a babyface. Approaching the gang of men with machetes, he stepped down from the bicycle, bowed his head, and spoke softly to them in their mother tongue. Mutai told them he was a schoolboy, trying to get home to his parents. A nearby off-duty policeman heard the exchange and intervened to persuade the men to let him through. Eventually, they did so.

Mutai walked on, head down, wheeling his bicycle. When the danger had passed, he remounted and sped home to his grandfather's farm. His family was shocked to see Geoffrey arrive from that direction. They told him the news: another Kalenjin boy had been killed in Timboroa the same day. Mutai felt a chill that has endured. The sight and smell of those burning houses remains vivid to him. "It was like a dream," he said. "It's not something I like to remember."

——

Mutai arrived into a world both ancient and modern. The eldest of Andrew and Emmy Koech's eleven children, he was born in a one-room, low-ceilinged, tin-roofed house in Equator, a village that sits at well over 8,000 feet of altitude, a mile or two south of the actual equator line.

In the first hours of Geoffrey's life, on the night of October 7, 1981, his grandparents called out the names of long-passed ancestors to soothe him, as was the custom of the Kipsigis. When one name was spoken by his grandmother, he stopped crying and sneezed—a sign that he had met his kindred spirit. Nobody in the family can now remember which ancestor's name caused the child to quit his bawling that night, and anyway, says Mutai, "I am a Christian. I don't believe in those traditions."

One part of his heritage, however, is inextinguishable. The Kipsigis are a subtribe of the Kalenjin, part of a Nilotic family of tribes who emerged from the Nile Valley centuries ago, and who now utterly dominate distance running.

In geographical terms, the Kalenjin are said to come from the "Rift Valley." But when people talk about the Rift Valley in Kenya, they can mean one of many things. The term refers both to a geological feature—the physical cleft in the earth's surface that divides Kenya west to east—and to a political entity that encompasses land stretching westward from the escarpment. Most often, the term is taken to mean the homelands of the Kalenjin: a high, lush, fertile land, good for farming.

This is a sticky topic. These lands were once Masai grazing territories, and Kikuyus have also settled in this territory. In the postelection violence of 2007–2008, in which Mutai found himself unintentionally embroiled, many observers interpreted the violence between Kikuyus and Kalenjin as a result not only of the political standoff, but as a by-product of an ongoing land dispute.

To make matters more complicated, the Kalenjin themselves are made up of further subtribes such as the Nandi, Keiyo, Kipsigis, Marakwet, and Pokot. Until the end of the British presence in Kenya in the 1960s, only two of these tribes lived permanently in the highlands: the Nandi and the Kipsigis, Mutai's group. The other subtribes lived in the valley, several thousand feet below, where it was warmer, and traveled up to the highlands a few times a year to graze their cattle. A significant number also worked for the colonials in the thin air. When the British left and a new land policy was enacted by the Kenyan government, the Kalenjin people from the valley were given the right to claim plots in the more fertile highlands. Most took the opportunity to settle above the escarpment.

This is a part of Kenya that tourists seldom visit. There are no game parks or beaches, no warriors in traditional dress performing for the cameras. But it's beautiful. The dominant colors are orange (the dirt roads, the sun) and green (the lush grass after a downpour, the bullrushes). Some of its views are indelible. Sitting on the western escarpment at Nyaru at sunset, you can see south and east for dozens of miles. Birds circle in the thermals near sharkstooth cliffs, and the shadows of high cloudlets dot the valley floor like spilled ink. You are reminded that this is the same valley from which, millennia ago, a group of men and women began their walk to all corners of the globe; the same valley from which the world's greatest runners have emerged.

Although the landscape is idyllic and the soil is rich, most people here are poor. They hustle. Visit Eldoret, the regional hub, where many of the most successful athletes, including Mutai, have bought expensive houses, and you get a sense of daily struggle. In the bustle and chaos, one is as likely to be overtaken by a donkey cart as by a pristine Japanese SUV. The place feels at once dilapidated and vital. Street kids sniff glue and beg money. You can buy pretty much anything, including knockoff Chinese car parts and synthetic erythropoietin—the hormone that boosts red blood cell production and has been at the center of recent doping scandals. Bars do a lively business.

There is a story about Eldoret's oldest bank, which is now the site of a branch of Barclays. The tale goes that when the first British settlers established themselves in Eldoret they decided they'd need somewhere to park their currency. So a thick safe was transported from Nairobi by cart. When it came to moving this safe from the cart, however, the men assigned to do so buckled under its weight. It slipped from their grasp and plunged into a boggy bit of ground. Seeing that it was going to be difficult to move the heavy metal from the mud, it was decided that the spot where the safe had landed was as good a place as any for the bank. The workers simply built bricks around the strongbox. The story—of which there are a couple of versions—may be an exaggeration. But whatever its veracity, the narrative tells its own truth. Eldoret is a make-do kind of town.

Although many runners have bought houses in Eldoret, almost all are country boys and girls from small villages. Mutai is no different. His grandfather Rakrui moved to Equator in the last days of colonial rule to work for a British family as a mechanic and odd-jobs man. When the British left, he stayed with his wife, Esther. Mutai's grandparents still work a farm about two miles from the small strip of shops on the main road. It's a gorgeous spot, high on a hillside, with fields yielding maize, potatoes, carrots, and cabbages. There is still no household electricity here, although Mutai is hoping to use his influence to have power lines installed.

Rakrui and Esther both have large holes in their earlobes, developed in their teens using earrings of ever-increasing size, as was the Kalenjin tradition. Esther also has delicate tattoos on her cheeks. Rakrui is now more than ninety years old and has worked long days for seventy years. His hearing is shot, he carries a walking stick, and he wears flimsy glasses that look like they've been fashioned out of an old coat hanger. But he still marches around the farm under his own steam, and scales fence stiles like a man half his age.

Mutai's grandfather is known in the village as the "the Muzungu": the white man. Obviously, he's not white. His grandson says he won the nickname not only because of his former employers, but because he began to exhibit a British stiff upper lip and sense of fair play.

"He is straight," Geoffrey explained. "You cannot hide anything from him. He is honest. If you come and complain to him, he says 'no.' He never wants lies."

——

Mutai says he was always happy in Equator. Despite the simplicity of his upbringing, he was certain of food, shelter, and love. He ran to and from his school, which was a few miles up the road. He played around the farm. His grandparents say that they adored him "like a son."

This blissful childhood, however, was sundered when Mutai's parents decided to move the family to a town called Rongai, which is many miles south of Equator, toward Nakuru. Soon afterward, his father lost his job at a textiles factory. The family struggled. There was no money to do anything other than survive. Mutai says that for a long period he couldn't sleep at home because there was not enough room in his father's house. Instead, he was taken in by neighbors.

The town of Rongai was a dead end—cursed, in Mutai's recollection, by the plague of alcoholism that infects swaths of rural Kenya. It was, Mutai remembers, "not good . . . There was no motivation there anymore. . . . When you finished school, you just stayed at home. Many of the young men there, they were drinking, drinking. Any guys that had talent lost it. If you are young there, you want only to marry and stay there. Not travel, not to do something else. When I go back there now, these men are begging me for money to drink."

Geoffrey traveled from Rongai to Equator at every opportunity, to stay with his grandparents. Eventually his parents would call him home. In this period, it wasn't just the lassitude of his contemporaries that bothered him, but his relationship with his father. Mutai said that his father, who was frustrated with his own lot, and angry at the world, had often beaten him. The infractions for which Geoffrey was punished were sometimes trivial. For instance, when he asked if he could build a small house for himself rather than relying on neighbors for shelter, his father sensed a challenge to his authority and disciplined him for his impudence. The beatings would sometimes become so vicious that Mutai fled to his grandparents. He never fought back. He always ran.

In his mid-teens, under these manifold pressures, Mutai started drinking with other boys his age. He remembers hazy, shameful mornings when he woke up in strange houses and did not know where he was. His schoolwork suffered. It took him four years longer than it should have to finish his primary education.

Despite and because of these strains, Mutai also discovered that he possessed a particular talent as a runner. There were few other Kalenjin boys at his school, and hardly any long-distance athletes. None of his classmates could understand why Geoffrey would want to flog himself round a track twenty-five times in a 10,000m race. But Mutai loved the *feel* of it, even when he ran alone. There was, he says, something "in his blood" to run.

At eighteen, having finally completed primary school and understanding that there was no money for further education, he returned to Equator, stayed with Rakrui, worked the farm, and lived clean. His grandfather gave him a small plot of land and encouraged him to build his own house on it. (That modest one-room cottage is still standing.) When Mutai lived in Rongai, he had thought, "This is the end of my life," but when he returned to his beloved grandparents, he saw possibilities. He began, in his words, "to focus."

In Equator, Mutai ran every morning, although he says now that he did not know his training sessions might blossom into a lucrative career. He says that he simply felt a joy in it—a pleasure connected to a childhood spent bounding up and down hills at the farm. (This recollection seems romantic at best. Mutai was an ambitious young man—he remembers seeing planes flying overhead and thinking, *one day*—and he must have known that athletic success might make him money. There was also at least one other professional athlete from his grandfather's village.)

In any event, Mutai says that money was never his main mo tivation. He remembers going to town to watch the 2000 Sydney Olympics on television, and catching Haile Gebrselassie's breath-stopping duel with Paul Tergat in the final of the 10,000m. As the two nonpareil runners of their generation fought each other to the tape in a stadium lit by dancing flashbulbs, Mutai recalls physically breaking out in sweats.

His training became more regular. By 2001, he was running with a friend named Josphat Keiyo, a soft-spoken, handsome man who still trains with Mutai. He began to compete in a few junior steeplechase and long-distance races with good results. The same year, he was selected for the Kenyan team bound for the African Junior Athletics Championships in Mauritius. But he could not travel to the games, on account of his not having a birth certificate. Mutai was devastated, but what could he do?

This was just one of many moments in which a career in running seemed to be beyond him. By 2005, when Mutai was in his early twenties, he had still not joined a regular training group and his progress had stalled. He thought about quitting the sport altogether. There were no athletes in the family and his parents were anxious for him to start out on a trade or business of some kind. When he sustained a serious injury to his calf, a friend managed to get him a job cutting trees and digging holes for Kenya Power: backbreaking work.

It was in this lowest period, however, that he became more convinced than ever that running should be his life. He remembers while working as a lumberjack watching another track meet on a barroom television and feeling the same as when he watched Tergat and Gebrselassie tear into one another in Sydney. "It was like . . . I feel I can fly," he said.

After his six-month contract with Kenya Power expired, and he was not given another job, he was adamant. He would somehow attach himself to a training group—any group—and make his ambition a reality.

———

Mutai found his way to Kapng'tuny, a tiny, desolate village that sits high in the hills to the southeast of the Burnt Forest in an area known as Skyline. The athletes call it "Skyland."

The village is a twenty-minute drive from the nearest tarmac road and sits nearly 9,000 feet above sea level. In colonial times, it used to be called Kapsasmith, after an Englishman named Smith who owned the homestead. Now Smith's old farmhouse is the primary school and the village has changed its name. The locals pronounce it "Kapen-ge-toon." It means "the place of the lions."

You're unlikely to see a lion. Things you will see: an unpaved, grassy main street, and two empty hotels with their windows smashed. The defunct establishments are called "Hotel Popular Joint" and "Fivestar Hotel." Other sights: a working *poshomill,* where maize is ground to make *ugali,* the starchy, sticky carbohydrate that fuels rural Kenya; a general convenience store, where you can buy a wrench or a Coke; and a generously stocked, fly-plagued butcher's shop. Nearby there is a simple restaurant that serves excellent *chapattis*—Indian-style pancakes that Kenyans often eat with their tea. In the afternoons, several working-age men wander into town from the surrounding countryside, aromatically drunk on *bus'aa* and *chang'aa*, the local hooch.

You will also see some of the world's greatest distance runners here. Skyland is a magical place to train—not too warm, even when sunny, and cold at night. It's higher than most training camps in Kenya and has dozens of miles of hard, rough roads and testing hills all around. Most important, it's remote. There are few distractions. The nearest big town, Eldoret, is an hour's drive away. In any event, most of the athletes don't have cars.

When Mutai joined the training group in Kapng'tuny it was led by a senior athlete named William Kiplagat, who had won marathons in Rotterdam and Amsterdam. The group had no coach. Unlike an increasing number of training groups in Kenyan running country that are administered and financed by European management groups, and employ professional coaches, the senior Kapng'tuny runners set their own programs. There was little dissent. Kiplagat had a personal best of 2:06:50 from the 1999 Amsterdam Marathon. At that time, remembers Mutai, "two-oh-six means you are a strong athlete." His program was the product of a century's worth of running wisdom.

———

Perhaps the most important new thinking in the area of long-distance training was done by the Finns in the early part of the twentieth century. The great Paavo Nurmi worked with his coach, Lauri Pihkala, to devise an effective pattern of interval training—interspersing periods of fast running with short breaks—as well as longer runs. Before this point, distance runners had mostly trained simply by running or walking distances at a steady pace.

The success of Nurmi's methods were self-evident: In an astonishing career, he defeated all comers at distances ranging from 1,500m to the marathon. He is the only man in history to have held the mile, 5,000m, and 10,000m world records at the same time.

The central planks of Nurmi's philosophy are still in existence today. The programs of the world's best runners contain a mixture of speedwork and long runs. But, while training has not changed in essence since the era of the Flying Finns, it has changed dramatically in degree and emphasis. These developments have come in waves. In the 1930s, the Swedish coach Gösta Holmer tweaked the Finnish interval training method and made it less standardized—a runner would alternate his pace over a run based on how he felt. This kind of interval work was eventually given the enduring name *Fartlek,* or "speedplay."

The great Czech champion Emil Zátopek took this idea to a new level, running a huge volume of high-intensity speedwork, sometimes in army boots and occasionally carrying his wife on his back to improve his strength—a method that failed to gain traction. Zátopek was not the prettiest athlete—he ran, in the words of one journalist, "like a man wrestling with an octopus on a conveyor belt"—but he was remarkably successful. At the 1952 Olympics he won three gold medals, in the 5,000m, 10,000m, and the marathon (in his first attempt at the distance).

In the 1950s and 1960s, the New Zealand coach Arthur Lydiard reversed Nurmi's philosophy and ensured that his runners gathered a huge "base" of miles before they even thought about speedwork. He believed it was imperative for elite runners to regularly tuck 100 miles a week under their belt, all run at sub-race pace. This trained the heart and the muscles for the rigors

of competition, whether the athlete was a champion 800m runner or a marathoner. Lydiard's approach has often been dubbed
LSD, for "long slow distance," but that's not quite an accurate
portrayal of his philosophy. His athletes would eventually inter-
sperse faster runs and hillwork with longer runs as their program progressed, but he wanted them to build from a huge base.

During the same era, the eccentric Australian coach Percy
Cerutty pioneered his "Stotan" approach (an ugly neologism
formed by combining "Stoic" and "Spartan"). He was obsessed
with running form, and his signature training technique was to
have his runners work on hills or in sand for "resistance training."
He also believed a runner needed a "strong trunk": core strength,
as we now understand it. Cerutty had some odd ideas—he didn't
believe in warming up, for instance—but his methods seemed to
work. His runners broke thirty world records.

The East African mentality is now a combination of Lydiard,
Zátopek, Nurmi, Cerutty, and their own homegrown philosophy.
Elite runners generally cover 120 miles or more during the week,
training at least twice a day for six days. There are variations on
this format. Some runners train three times a day when they are
building their mileage base. Some train on Sundays. All of them
sleep an extraordinary number of hours a day. (Lornah Kiplagat
swears by sixteen hours' sleep a day when she is in full training.)
Very few do any work in the gym to build core strength. They are
conditioned by running alone.

The Kenyan system is designed to simultaneously build speed
and endurance. A favorite Kenyan workout is the "progression
run," a long-distance training session that starts slow and finishes at a rapid pace. But what really distinguishes the modern
marathon elite from their forebears is the large volume of high-

intensity work that they do. It is now common for the best athletes to complete a single speedwork session covering 2,000m ten times (a total of 20km, nearly a half marathon's worth of work). The men who make money at the marathon are now *fast*. Whereas marathoners of the past might have struggled at shorter distances on the track, most of the current generation of champions could all have had excellent careers at 5,000m.

———

In Kapng'tuny, Mutai found the cheapest accommodation he could and trained his guts out. Most of the time, he was broke. Life was not easy. But he refused to let material privations deter him. He remembers telling himself: "Nobody was born with anything. Your father was not born with anything. Get up. Work."

The camp was more than twenty miles away from Equator. When weekends came, Mutai walked there and back—even in the rainy season when the mud was thigh-high in places. He soon moved into shared accommodation with other junior athletes. One of the bedrooms he lived in during this period was directly outside the front door of Kapng'tuny's only nightclub, a tin-roofed sweatbox called Club 2000. On the weekends, he made money by selling vegetables from the family farm. Every cent he earned was spent on rent and food. Throughout this difficult period, he held a prayer in his head: "Please God, one day my time will come."

Patience: the word means both to wait and to suffer. In his first months in Kapng'tuny, Mutai would need to do both. He still carried injuries that had plagued him in his early twenties. His parents continued to badger him to give up the sport. He was unwavering, but running began to seem more like a plight than a destiny. Sometimes at night he cried as he lay in bed because his body could not keep pace with his ambition.

But alongside these pressures, there was the simple pleasure of running with a group of forty or fifty other men, two or three times a day: the fellowship, the jokes, the nicknames, the advice. In the long interstices between training sessions they would sun bathe and swap stories over cups of chai. These colleagues, in Mutai's remembrance, became his brothers.

By 2007, after two years of following a regular program, Mutai's shape improved. He could now keep pace with the strongest men in Kapng'tuny. When he heard about a road race near his home village, he entered and won. With the bicycle he received as first prize, he could compete in events that could not be reached on foot. He also met a girl from his village that year, a sweet, taciturn woman named Beatrice, whom he married. And at the end of the year he entered the Kass Marathon in Eldoret, a prestigious event closely watched by European managers.

Mutai remembers waking up in Eldoret on the day of the race with some other athletes who had traveled from Kapng'tuny and finding nowhere open for breakfast. It was well before dawn. Eventually they discovered a man selling tea and bread on the street. The other athletes were skeptical of the street vendor, believing that his products would make them ill, but Mutai insisted. He argued persuasively that if they wouldn't eat from the street vendor they wouldn't eat at all. It proved a wise decision. They saw nowhere else to eat before boarding the official bus to the startline of the race.

Hours later, with a little food in his belly, Mutai ran an outstanding debut at altitude—2 hours and 12 minutes—which was good enough for second place. A Dutch manager named Gerard

Van de Veen was watching. By his side was a gregarious athlete Van de Veen represented named Wilson Kigen, who was also a member of Mutai's Skyland training group.

"This is my boy!" Kigen hollered to Van de Veen as Mutai flew by in second place.

Van de Veen was impressed. It wasn't just that Mutai had performed well in the race, but he possessed an easy, efficient style. It was the start of Mutai's professional relationship with his Dutch manager. They signed a contract the day after the race. Van de Veen, who had seen that Mutai was good on hills, booked him to run the Monaco Marathon, a mountainous course, in March 2008.

"That was the day," Mutai said of the Kass Marathon. "My life started there."

——

His life almost finished a month later at the hands of the mob in Timboroa. Once the shock of that incident had subsided, Mutai became angry. He had worked so hard for his opportunity at the Kass Marathon and had found himself a manager who could help him race for serious money. Now the country was in turmoil. Hundreds of people were dying, and hundreds of thousands were displaced from their homes. What Kenyans referred to euphemistically as "postelection" had arrived, and with it perhaps Mutai's chances of fulfilling his talent had departed.

Even training became dangerous. On long runs, the athletes didn't know whom they would meet. The marathon runner Wesley Ngetich was killed during the violence by a poison arrow. The world marathon champion Luke Kibet was severely injured when he was struck by a stone.

The violence eventually abated. On February 28, 2008, Mwai Kibaki and Raila Odinga, the two rival politicians at the center of the postelection crisis, signed a power-sharing agreement. Although his training had been interrupted by Kenya's convulsions, Mutai would travel to Monaco and compete in his first outside marathon. He became giddy with excitement.

Everything was new to him. First of all, he needed to take three flights to reach Monaco. He had never been on a plane before. Mutai remembers reaching the small terminal at Eldoret airport and becoming worried that there were too many people to fit on his flight to Nairobi. He had only ever seen planes from the ground, and at that distance, they seemed impossibly small. Now there were dozens of people around him in the terminal— too many, he calculated, for everyone to get a seat. Worried that the last arrivers would not be admitted, he pushed his way to the front of the line to board.

Then there was the landing of his final flight, at Nice Côte d'Azur Airport. The runway sits on a spit on the southern coast of France. As his plane made its final approach over the Mediterranean Sea, Mutai remembers entertaining the prospect that he might land in the water and prepared himself for a bump and splash.

And then there was Monaco itself. Mutai found the place ridiculous. People in Monaco drove their cars in tunnels and treated their dogs in hospitals. The houses were all piled up on the hillside. Even the Louis II soccer stadium, where the marathon finished, was somehow resting on top of another building. Mutai laughed himself silly. "How did they build those houses?" he remembers thinking. "How did they make that place look like that? It was unbelievable!"

As the race approached, Mutai felt primed. He refused to carry any heaviness from the postelection violence, or his many years of struggle, or his unhappy adolescence. Here he was, in this odd place where rich *muzungus* lived crushed together, and he had a chance to change his fortunes.

On the day of the marathon, Van de Veen was there to assist him. His manager watched the race from the pace truck. In Van de Veen's recollection, Mutai made the mountainous course, out and back to Ventimiglia in Italy, look easy. He ran steady for the first half, then pushed twice—once at 30km, and again at 35km. In doing so, he smoked his competitors, who had the historic misfortune to race a debutant at the beginning of an outstanding career. Mutai won the race in 2:12:40. The prize money was 4,000 euros. His life as an international athlete had begun.

Chapter Four

Bright Lights, Big Cities

1976, 1896, and all that

T HE SPORT that Mutai entered in Monaco—professional city
marathoning—began its life only thirty-two years earlier, on
a cool, bright morning in Manhattan, when a good-looking, rail-
thin American with bouncing blond hair galloped into Central
Park. It was lunchtime on October 24, 1976. The man's name was
Bill Rodgers, and the race he was about to win was the inaugural
five-borough New York City Marathon.

As Rodgers came into the park, taking his last few hundred
steps toward the finish at the Tavern on the Green, the crowd
was a dozen deep in places and pressing the course. He was
wearing a white Greater Boston vest, red shorts, and white
gloves like a butler. Behind him, spectators riding bicycles
took a close-up look. In the scrum, a town car that had been
leading the way got snagged, and Rodgers was forced to dodge

around it. He'd been doing a lot of dodging over the past two hours and nine minutes: running up and down steps, slogging over bridges, leaping potholes. The course, he thought, was like urban cross-country.

The finish line was marked by a banner that looked like it had been fashioned at home, and was held up by two volunteers. By the time Rodgers ran beneath it—hands up in a spirit of "don't shoot" rather than "champion of the world"—the canvas had already started to sag in the middle. In the seconds after Rodgers recorded a winning time of 2:10:10, he shook one hand, and then another, and had his picture taken a dozen times. He soaked up the attention, a toothy smile on his face, like a startled squirrel.

Rodgers had many reasons to be happy. Not only was he the champion of the first city-wide New York marathon, he was also the first *professional* winner of the race. Unbeknownst to most onlookers, who believed in the sport's amateur status, Rodgers had been paid three thousand dollars in appearance money to run in New York City. It wasn't much, but it was something.

The 1976 New York race was the first time a major city marathon in America had enticed its star runners with appearance fees. Despite strict rules laid down by the sport's governing bodies that athletes should not be remunerated, both Rodgers and his rival, the Olympic gold medalist Frank Shorter, were paid to join battle in New York. It proved a watershed for the sport. In the years following the 1976 New York City Marathon, it became clear that the old rules were unsustainable. Clandestine appearance money became normal for marathoners, and then acceptable. In 2013, the British runner Mo Farah was reported to have been paid more than a million dollars to compete in the London Marathon.

There is a view that the marathon, one of the founding Olympic disciplines, has been spoiled by money—that "Dollar Bill" Rodgers and his contemporaries somehow corrupted it with their grubby demands. You can see the remnants of that Corinthian outlook in the vestigial amateurism that exists in the marathon today. This is a sport in which the amounts of appearance money paid to athletes is still a closely held secret. As Mary Wittenberg, CEO of New York Road Runners, admitted in 2013: "Somehow the word 'professional' has turned into a bad word."

It was not always a bad word. In fact, in asking for money to compete, Bill Rodgers was connecting to a much deeper history of the sport than the rulemakers acknowledged. Even before the first modern Olympic Games in 1896—when the marathon made its first official amateur outing there was money in the race. By tracing the story of professionalism in the marathon, you can draw a direct line between the early history of the race, its revolution in the 1970s, and the current generation of pioneers who now climb higher and higher toward the sport's mountaintop.

———

There is no better creation myth in sports. In 490 BC, a Greek named Pheidippides was sent to seek help from the Spartan army when the Persians landed near Marathon, Greece. Pheidippides was a *hemerodromos,* a professional long-distance running courier, and his feats of endurance were prodigious. First, he is said to have run 150 miles in two days in order to fetch help. Then he ran about 25 miles, from the battlefield near Marathon to Athens, to proclaim a Greek victory. According to Lucian, the writer who first narrated this tale, Pheidippides proclaimed to the expectant Athenian worthies "Chairete, Nikomen!" ("Joy to you, we've won!") before dying on the spot from exhaustion.

This story passed into lore. Plutarch wrote a similar tale in which the runner's name was Euclus or Thersippus. (The details were essentially identical: man completes long run, proclaims victory, expires.) The tale lay largely dormant until the nineteenth century, when Pheidippides became the subject of creative attention once more. In 1834, a statue of the runner by the French sculptor Cortot was erected in the Tuileries Garden in Paris. Then, in 1879, Robert Browning wrote a poem about Pheidippides in which he killed off the messenger at his moment of triumph in the following purple tones:

> Yes, he fought on the Marathon day:
> So, when Persia was dust, all cried "To Akropolis!
> Run, Pheidippides, one race more! The meed is thy due!
> 'Athens is saved, thank Pan,' go shout!" He flung down his shield,
> Ran like fire once more: and the space 'twixt the Fennel-field
> And Athens was stubble again, a field which a fire runs through,
> Till in he broke: "Rejoice, we conquer!" Like wine thro' clay,
> Joy in his blood bursting his heart, he died—the bliss!

Sometime in the next decade, a French philologist named Michel Bréal read Browning's poem and had an idea. His friend Baron de Coubertin was in the process of organizing the first modern Olympics, to be held in Athens in 1896. In 1894, on the suggestion of Bréal, Coubertin proposed a "Marathon race" as part of the Olympic program to celebrate Pheidippides's feat and tragic demise.

No matter that the Pheidippides marathon story was bunk.

Lucian was a satirist, not a historian, and his account of the messenger's heroic run from Marathon to Athens appears to be a conflation of various other narratives. Moreover, Lucian's story only appeared for the first time in the second century AD. There is no contemporary record of the feat, nor is there any mention made of the Marathon-to-Athens run by Herodotus, the Greek "father of history," in his account of the battle.

However, according to Herodotus, at least one part of the myth is correct. Not only was there a *hemerodromos* involved in the battle, but his feats appear to have been the genesis for an annual running race. Herodotus writes that a runner named Philippides was dispatched to deliver a message from Athens to Sparta to seek help in fighting the approaching Persian army. The Spartans demurred. Philippides covered a distance of 135–155 miles over mountainous terrain in less than two days: an extraordinary endeavor, undertaken in vain. Herodotus adds that in the Parthenian mountains, the messenger encountered the god Pan, who asked him why the Athenians no longer threw parties in his honor. When Philippides related this message to the people of Athens, the worthies of that city decreed that a torchlit race, and a feast, be held for Pan.

The origin of the Marathon-to-Athens myth, meanwhile, most likely lies in the forced march the Athenian troops made over that ground in the hours following their victory against the Persians. After their victory on the battlefield at Marathon, the Greek generals were concerned that the Persian navy could attack Athens from the west. So the army slogged back to the capital that same day: more than twenty miles, in full armor. This march appears to have been achieved in around six or seven hours—another impressive feat of athleticism, but not the one Browning sold us.

—

The organizers of the first Olympics were not keen to let facts ruin a good story. On April 10, 1896, they got their marathon race. It was the final event of the Games in which the Greeks had not won a thing. And, although the first Olympics had been designed by Coubertin to promote amateur ideals and a Corinthian spirit, there was a certain amount of pressure on the home team to produce a victory. The main financial backer of the Games, a Greek businessman named Georgios Averoff, is said to have offered a tempting reward for any local man to cross the finish line in first place: his daughter's hand in marriage and a million-drachma dowry.

At 2 p.m. on a warm Friday, eighteen men toed the startline of the 25-mile course. Fourteen of the starters were Greek. But it was a Frenchman, Albin Lermusiaux, running in white gloves in honor of the Greek king, who set the early pace. At a little after the 9-mile mark he was more than a mile ahead of the chasing pack. By the time he reached the town of Karvati, he was so far ahead of his competitors that the locals put a wreath of victory on his head. He accepted their attentions. The Greeks have a word for this sort of behavior: *hubris.*

At 19 miles the Frenchman became the first man in the history of the Olympic marathon to "hit the wall." His legs went to jelly. He was overtaken by Teddy Flack, an Australian. (Flack was accompanied and assisted by the British ambassador's butler, who rode a bicycle alongside him.) A mile or so later, Flack was joined by a Greek named Spyridon Louis, who had paced his race adroitly and looked fresh.

At around this time, it is said, Louis was handed some slices of orange by a girl he would later marry. (This story, for which there is a single contemporary source, may also be a product of the myth factory.) Whatever happened to Louis in the closing stages of the race, he ran like a *hemerodromos* on a mission. As Louis found new strength, Flack faded so badly he would be taken to the finish line in an ambulance wagon.

When Louis entered the marble stadium, thronged with 60,000 spectators, a cannon was fired. Crown Prince Constantine and Prince George of Greece were so thrilled at the arrival of a Greek in first place that they ran a full circuit of the running track with the victor-elect before he crossed the line in 2 hours, 58 minutes, and 50 seconds: the first sub-three-hour marathon. At the victory ceremony, Louis was awarded a silver medal and a wreath of olive branches. He turned down Averoff's offer of his daughter's hand in marriage. It was reported, however, that he did accept free meals and haircuts for life, as well as a new horse and cart from the king, to replace his donkey. He never ran competitively again.

———

The broadly accepted history of the sport says that Spyridon Louis's victory was the spark that lit the flame of modern marathon running. The story goes that, after the Greek Olympiad, spectators who had watched Louis's triumph spread the gospel of the marathon far and wide.

That narrative, however, does not hold water. It's true that a group of Americans watching the race on April 10, 1896, returned to Boston and established the oldest continuously contested marathon in the world—an event where, 115 years after that sunny day in Athens, the performance of Geoffrey Mutai would cause people to reconsider what kind of an event the marathon really was. It's also true that without the Athens race and its ensuing Olympic journey, the marathon as we know it today—the eccentric 26-mile, 385-yard race—would not exist.

But people ran "marathons" before the Olympics existed. And they ran for money long before they ran for long-dead Greeks. In England, there are reports of endurance races taking place between the servants of rich men as early as the seventeenth century. Sometimes their rich employers would wager on the outcome, and sometimes the workingmen needed no such encouragement. The diarist Samuel Pepys records several instances of "foot-races" in London, including this note from Friday, August 10, 1660: "I went and dined at home, and after dinner with great pain in my back I went by water to Whitehall to the Privy Seal, and that done with Mr. Moore and Creed to Hide Park by coach, and saw a fine foot-race three times round the Park between an Irishman and Crow, that was once my Lord Claypoole's footman. . . . Crow beat the other by above two miles."

A full circuit of Hyde Park is now around five miles, and the park has shrunk since Pepys's day. Crow and the Irishman appear to have run the best part of a marathon for sport.

"Pedestrianism"—a catchall term for running and walking—gained popularity in the nineteenth century. Indeed, before that first Olympic Games in 1896, there had been a lively professional distance running scene in both America and Europe. For instance, on the east coast of America, in the early part of the nineteenth century, blue-collar athletes would challenge each other to footraces of anything up to 12 miles for a set purse and whatever they could make in side bets. Sometimes a promoter would advertise a cash prize for any runner beating a certain time.

Such races were not only well paid but energetically supported. In June 1835, a field of nine runners assembled on the startline on the Union Course in Long Island to win a purse of $1,300 for anyone completing 10 miles in less than an hour. Between 16,000 and 20,000 spectators turned out to watch, and the road from Brooklyn to the Union Course was said to be a solid line of carriages "from the humble sand car to the splendid barouche and four." The race organizer, a Mr. Stevens, apparently became so terrified at the sums of money being wagered that he announced he was postponing the event. When his decision nearly provoked a riot, he promptly reversed it, and the race went ahead.

As the athletes made their way around the track, a trumpet was blasted every six minutes to show the spectators whether the runners were behind, or in front of, a one-hour pace (an ingenious strategy that today's marathon promoters might do well to copy). One of the competitors, Henry Stannard, was shrewd enough to employ a pacer on horseback, who trotted alongside him to ensure he kept to his race plan—and, sure enough, Stannard prevailed. He was the only man to break one hour. The final trumpet that sounded twelve seconds after he crossed the line could not be heard above the cheering of the crowd.

In Britain, meanwhile, races were being held between professionals over what we would now describe as a "marathon" distance. The British track historian Andy Milroy argues that professional pedestrians had been competing at 25 miles for most of the nineteenth century. It was, he writes, the "standard distance." In 1824, for instance, Robert Skipper, the "Champion of England," was challenged to a match over "25 miles of ground."

Two decades later, professional contests of this length had become common. On May 23, 1844, the *Times* of London reported on one of these 25-mile races.

GREAT FOOT RACE—The anxiously-looked for and long-talked of great pedestrian match between George Bradshaw, of Hammersmith, and B. Butler, of Hanwell, came off on Tuesday at Smitham Bottom. Both men are great favorites with the public, and may be assuredly looked upon as the two greatest pedestrians of this or of any antecedent period. Bradshaw signalized himself a few months ago in a match of 25 miles with the celebrated Robert Fuller, whom he defeated, after a struggle never surpassed, and in which his speed, style, and unflinching game were so fully established, that his friends selected a customer for him in the person of Butler, who had within three years beaten all before him. . . . Butler had never before been engaged in a 25 mile race, and therefore his time at that distance was unknown to the public, while Bradshaw had on the other hand accomplished it, in his race with Fuller, under four hours. . . . The assemblage of spectators on the ground was immense, and included many good sporting men. Shortly after 2 o'clock the pedestrians made their appearance, and a greater disparity between rival walkers we never remember to have seen. Butler is about six feet two, and a very powerful man with it, while his opponent does not appear to exceed five feet eight, and is very thin and spare; it was what in sporting phraseology might be termed "a horse to a hen." The men did not get away until half-past

2, when they effected a very beautiful start; and, although the race in-flicted a severe disappointment upon the multitude who had travelled so far to witness it, the early part was evenly and beautifully con-tested. For the first eight miles and a half the men were shoulder and shoulder, with the exception of a trifling spurt or so, of which the first two miles were done in 17 minutes, and the six miles in 53 minutes. The greatest excitement prevailed on all hands. It was considered to be anybody's victory, and money was being laid out from the seventh to the eighth mile very freely. After turning the eighth mile, it was evident to those acquainted with such matters that Bradshaw was giving way, and before their arrival at the ninth milestone he relaxed his speed, and Butler went ahead. From this moment it looked, and was, a dead certainty, Butler increased his advantage in every step, and in the 15th mile Bradshaw, having struggled on until then with a violent pain in the side, as it was declared, resigned. Butler took it very comfortably the remainder of the distance, and completed the 25 miles in four hours and a half. He had been trained by the great and highly respectable pedestrian, Temperance, who attended upon him during the race.

These early races over more than 20 miles would normally have been contested by walkers rather than runners. For a long time, it was considered folly to run so far. But in the second half of the century, something strange happened to pedestrian-ism. The highest-profile pedestrian contests grew monstrous in length and profile. They became ultra-endurance events that sometimes lasted as long as six days, over hundreds of miles, and took place in packed, smoke-filled halls, for huge cash prizes—and were guarded by dozens of policemen to stop bettors from interfering with the athletes.

With the advent of this ultra-endurance pedestrianism, many professional races became "go-as-you-please," a technique mixing walking and running, rather than the stricter "fair-heel-and-toe" rule. This development led to out-and-out running over distances of about 25 miles. By the 1870s and 1880s, professional runners in Britain, Sweden, Germany, France, and Italy began to turn in impressive performances at what is now, roughly, a marathon length.

The best result from these pioneering "marathons" was achieved in England by an amateur named George Dunning. With acute pacing, he achieved a world record time of 2 hours, 33 minutes, and 44 seconds for 25 miles, at the Stamford Bridge track on Boxing Day, 1881. This record stood for 22 years until Len Hurst—one of the early professional stars of distance running and the first winner of the Paris Marathon in 1896—broke it at the Tee-To-Tum ground in Stamford Hill, London, in 1903.

As a standard distance, 25 miles makes sense because it neatly tallies with a round number of 40 kilometers in the metric system. The historian Andy Milroy also suggests that a 25-mile race might have been attractive to the organizers of the first Olympics as it was the only long distance at which the world record was held by an amateur runner. But whatever the specific origins of the Olympic marathon, the event was as much a product of the existing professional distance-running circuit as it was a recreation of an ancient Greek myth.

——

After the triumph of the 1896 race in Athens, the Olympic marathon went into a slump. At the 1900 Paris Olympics, the marathon was poorly organized and marred by accusations of cheating. In temperatures that peaked at over 100 degrees, only 7 of the 13 starters—from five countries—finished the course. The gold medal was won by Michel Théato, representing France, in a little under three hours. Soon after his victory, the American delegation accused Théato of taking shortcuts. They said that, as a Parisian baker, he would know every side street and back alley in the city. In fact, Théato was not a baker but a cabinetmaker— and he was not even French, having been born in Luxembourg. There is no evidence he cheated.

At the calamitous 1904 Olympics in St. Louis, however, the organizers of the marathon race needed no proof to see that their winner had bent the rules. He confessed.

The entire event was a grisly shambles. On a stinking hot August day in Missouri, on dusty roads, a caravan of vehicles progressed ahead of the field, kicking up a throat-coating sand- storm. Of the 32 entrants, only 14 finished the race. So appalling were the conditions that one contestant ruptured his esophagus before halfway.

In a field in which all but four athletes represented America, a five-foot Cuban postman named Andarín Carvajal, who wore a beret and cutoff trousers, led the field until well past halfway. The legend has it that, in the closing stages of the race, having not eaten for forty hours, Carvajal raided an orchard for apples and was subsequently struck down by stomach cramps. This may or may not be true. There is a record of Carvajal stealing peaches from a reporter covering the race, but recently, the historian George R. Matthews has questioned the orchard story. In any event, the Cuban finished fourth.

Fred Lorz, a New York bricklayer, had endured enough dust and misery by nine miles, and hopped in a car. He only got out of the vehicle at the 20-mile mark, when the car broke down. As John Bryant relates in *The Marathon Makers,* Lorz then jogged the remaining distance to the stadium, which he entered looking "strangely cool" and where he was feted as the winner. He played along for a while, running a victory lap and having his picture taken with President Theodore Roosevelt's oldest daughter, Alice. Shortly afterward, he admitted to his practical joke and was disqualified. After the Olympics, Lorz was banned from athletics. Having served his one-year suspension, he won the 1905 Boston Marathon under his own steam.

The real victor, Thomas Hicks from Massachusetts, was propelled to the finish line by a cocktail of brandy, egg whites, and strychnine—otherwise known as rat poison. He finished the race like a puppet with its strings cut. There is a photograph of him, shortly after he had been resuscitated by doctors in the stadium, that is among the more terrifying sporting images you could ever wish to see. Hicks is sitting at the wheel of an automobile, surrounded by a gaggle of his serious-looking supporters. His face is wan, and his eyes are sunken. He looks half dead—which is what, by contemporary accounts, he was.

Amid this chicanery, one story from that unlovely day in 1904 pointed toward the distant future of the sport. Two men who represented South Africa in the event were black Tswana tribesmen from the Orange Free State named Len Tau and Jan Mashiani. By running the marathon that day, they became the first black Africans to compete in the Olympics.

Tau and Mashiani were in St. Louis as part of a repulsive "cultural" sideshow at the World's Fair—a program of "athletic events for savages" that included rock throwing and tree climbing. In the Olympic marathon, however, they competed with aplomb.

Mashiani finished twelfth and Tau ninth, and it was reported that Tau would have finished much faster had he not lost precious minutes being chased a mile off course by an aggressive dog.

After 1904, the marathon was in dire shape. Having watched the finish of both the Paris and St. Louis marathons, James Sullivan—the director of the first American Olympic Games—questioned the sanity of allowing the race to continue, saying that he believed the distance to be "man-killing in effect." He went so far as to convene a committee to discuss the future of the discipline. No record of any meeting exists, but if one took place, its conclusions are evident: the marathon survived.

By the time the Olympics reached London in 1908, however, the wisdom and entertainment value of watching a group of men struggle over such a long distance still seemed questionable. Another debacle like St. Louis or Paris might have relegated the marathon race to the scrapheap of short-lived Olympic sports— a dishonor that has since been bestowed upon such events as the tug-of-war and Basque pelota. It was good fortune for all of us, then, that the 1908 Olympic marathon was one of the most wonderful and controversial races of all time.

———

The course of the London Olympic marathon of 1908 was 26 miles and 385 yards long—a peculiar distance that comes with its own mythology attached. Before this time, "marathons" had been run at any distance around 25 miles, but the organizers of the London games were anxious to gain the royal family's approval. They wanted to begin the race at Windsor Castle and have it finish beneath the royal box in the White City stadium. Jack Andrew, a member of the Polytechnic Harriers club who designed the 1908 marathon, said that their initial suggestion for a course fulfilling these criteria was 24 and a half miles. But the Harriers tinkered with their design when they realized that a professional race intended to use the same route.

The organizers eventually decided on a course of around 26 miles that was designed to begin underneath the East Terrace of Windsor Castle so that the royal family's children could watch the start. It was stretched further by adding a full circuit of the track in the stadium to show off the athletes before they finished beneath the royal box. With these adjustments, the final distance for the race on July 24, 1908, was advertised as "around 26 miles and three hundred and eighty-five yards." ("Around" may be right. John Disley, one of the cofounders of the modern London Marathon, found the first "mile" of the 1908 course to be 174 yards short.)

There were 55 starters at the 1908 Olympic marathon, representing sixteen nations. Among these contenders, the reigning Boston marathon champion, a Canadian man from the native Onondaga tribe named Tom Longboat, was considered a favorite. According to John Bryant's history of the marathon, when Longboat arrived in Windsor for the start of the race, he saw a crowd of Eton schoolboys in their top hats and tails, and quipped, "Where's the funeral?"

The funeral was nearly his. Longboat collapsed well before the finish line. The race instead became a three-way contest between Charles Hefferon, a prison officer from South Africa; Dorando Pietri, a confectioner from Carpi, in Italy; and Johnny Hayes, an American subway tunneler who had recently become a Bloomingdale's employee.

Hayes is reported to have remarked to a fellow competitor at the startline, "It's hot, there's a long, long way to go, don't go crazy." He knew what he was talking about. Hayes's life to that point had been tough. A second-generation Irish immigrant to New York, he was orphaned when his parents died within two weeks of each other. There was no money for headstones; his younger siblings were taken in by a Catholic orphanage. Soon after, Hayes became a "sandhog"—digging tunnels for the New York subway—which was hotter work than a run from Windsor to London, whatever the weather.

Running freed Hayes from this low-paid drudgery. Members of the Irish American Athletic Club in Queens, like Hayes, were often found honorary "jobs" by their Hibernian brethren so that they would have time to train. Some athletes joined the New York Police Department, but Hayes, at five feet, four inches, was too small to work as a cop. In 1905, the IAAC found him a position at Bloomingdale's. Records don't exist of whether he actually turned up to work, but we do know that he trained on the store's rooftop cinder track at night. This new arrangement had a propulsive effect on his running career. In the years following his retirement from tunneling, he finished on the podium at the Yonkers and Boston marathons.

Like Hayes, Pietri hung back in the early stages. The Italian was a veteran of long-distance races in hot weather in Italy, and he wore a handkerchief doused in balsamic vinegar on his head that he would occasionally put in his mouth to refresh himself. As he ran, he repeated a mantra under his breath—*vincero o moriro*: win or die.

At the front of the field, the lead swapped a few times before

Hefferon, the South African, took control of the race at 15 miles and established a firm advantage. With two miles to go, Hefferon faltered when he accepted a glass of champagne from a spectator ("the drink gave me a cramp," he later told reporters). Pietri overtook him with an injection of speed. Hayes, a good distance back from Pietri, overtook Hefferon soon afterward. This spurt, however, appears to have destroyed Pietri, and by the time he reached the stadium, which was packed with around 90,000 spectators, he was spent. He turned the wrong way onto the track, before righting himself, and then collapsing.

Sir Arthur Conan Doyle, the author of the Sherlock Holmes novels, was covering the marathon for the *Daily Mail*. His report captures Pietri's dramatic attempt to finish the race in vivid detail:

> Good Heavens, he has fainted; is it possible that even at this last moment the prize may slip through his fingers? Every eye slides round to that dark archway. No second man has yet appeared. Then a sigh of relief goes up. I do not think in all that great assembly any man would have wished victory to be torn at the last instant from this plucky little Italian. . . . Thank God, he is on his feet again—the little red legs going incoherently, but drumming hard, driven by a supreme will. There is a groan as he falls once more, and a cheer as he staggers to his feet.

After one too many falls, Michael Bulger, the medical officer of the race, intervened. The doctor massaged Pietri's chest to keep his heart beating. But after each collapse, Pietri would rise seconds later and stagger a few more yards. By the final stages, Pietri was being assisted by both Bulger and Jack Andrew, the secretary of the race. One fall happened right in front of Conan

Doyle, who wrote, "I caught a glimpse of the haggard, yellow face, the glazed expressionless eyes. Surely he is done now?"

As Hayes entered the stadium in second place, the crowd roared and a brass band played "The Conquering Hero." Pietri was still 20 yards or so from the line. Andrew and Bulger all but carried the little Italian as he crested the tape—a moment of heroism and chaos famously captured in a remarkable shot by an unknown photographer from the Topical Press Agency. Pietri appeared to have won the race but was soon disqualified for receiving assistance from the officials, after an appeal by the Americans. Hayes was subsequently named the winner. The decision was unpopular. Pietri himself complained that he could have reached the finish line under his own steam. But the next day, justice was seen to be done when the Italian was awarded a silver gilt cup by the Queen in recognition of his courage.

Having read the newspaper reports of the great race in London, the world was suddenly ablaze for the marathon. The athletes sniffed a commercial opportunity. Pietri traveled to New York City to contest the race everybody wanted to see: Hayes versus Pietri II. Of course, the race would be contested over the "London distance" that had so nearly finished off Pietri: 26 miles and 385 yards. The American promoters also decided that they would hold the race inside, at Madison Square Garden, and sell tickets.

The rematch, which was held on November 25, 1908, was a sellout. Hayes and Pietri ran 262 laps of a track inside the old Garden in a bear-pit atmosphere. A journalist from the *New York Times* described the atmosphere at "the most spectacular foot race that New York has ever witnessed":

The immense hall was filled completely when the race was finished, with an attendance that included every class, from the gallery gods to the patrons of first nights and grand opera, and partisan feeling swayed the enormous gathering with such force that the rival brass bands, one of Italian musicians for Pietri, whom the crowd insistently called by his first name, and who thus popularly became Dorando, and another band, that of the Sixty-ninth Regiment, for the Irish-American athlete, were drowned in the clamor.

Flags waved and partisans cheered until the big amphitheater trembled with sound, and through it all the rival runners plodded around the ten-laps-to-the-mile track, and inhaled the dust and tobacco smoke with which the hall reeked in their reproduction of their struggle over twenty-six miles and 385 yards of English road in the Summer air of last June [*sic*].

At the conclusion of the race, which Pietri won, the *Times* reported that a riot was "narrowly averted."

——

Marathon mania had arrived in America. It would soon spread to Europe and Canada. For the next two years, contests between long-distance runners would sell out halls in New York, London, and Montreal. One race between Pietri and the Englishman C. W. Gardiner, which took place at London's Royal Albert Hall in December 1909, was particularly surreal. As the athletes ran in tiny circles on a 90-yard track made of coconut matting, the spectators listened to an Italian tenor who had been booked by the promoters to make the time pass "more pleasantly." Gardiner won the 524-lap race in 2 hours and 37 minutes. Dorando retired in the 482nd lap with blisters.

For Pietri, marathon mania must have been exhausting. He ran 22 races in the six months that began with the first Madison Square Garden rematch against Hayes, many of them at "the London distance." He won 17 of them. (His brother and manager, Ulpiano, who claimed 50 percent of his earnings, was behind this sadistic schedule.)

By 1910, however, the marathon fire had fizzled, in America at least. A San Francisco journalist, Franklin B. Morse, reported that the final "re-match" between Hayes and Pietri in his hometown contained all the excitement of watching "two old ladies engaged in a long-distance knitting contest." But before the guttering of the craze, several important things had happened to the marathon event. Most significant, its parameters had been set. The London distance of 26 miles, 385 yards was now considered standard and would be enshrined as the official length by the International Olympic Committee in 1921.

Moreover, the public and athletes alike started to consider where the limits of human endurance might lie. There was one unusual event in the short-lived marathon craze that has gone mostly unnoticed in standard histories of the sport. It was a "team race" over the marathon distance, contested by pairs of athletes, who each ran consecutive half miles. The race was held at Madison Square Garden on November 29, 2010, and featured five teams, from America, Finland, Canada, England, and a French-Swedish duo. The English team included Alf Shrubb, holder of the world one-hour run record, and the Finnish team the future Olympic marathon winner, Hannes Kolehmainen, who was noted for the silky smoothness of his stride. But it was the American pair, Hans Holmer and William Queal, who produced the most electrifying performance. They ran 13 miles in

58:55, meaning they ran a sub-one-hour first half. In the second half, they slowed only slightly, finishing in 2 hours, 2 minutes, and 16 seconds.

There is no record of another team marathon of this kind taking place anywhere in the world, after this remarkable event at the Garden. The indoor marathon relay record remains Holmer and Queal's—stranded 136 seconds from the magic two-hour mark.

——

By the 1950s, the marathon had reverted to a minor amateur pursuit sustained by the Olympic Games, and—in America—by the yearly pleasure of watching a small group of athletes compete in the Boston and Yonkers marathons. Nobody at those races got paid to run. Even in the 1960s, when the number of road races began to multiply, long-distance running carried a strange reputation. It was a niche activity, for oddballs and hippies. As Bill Rodgers remembers, America only understood "short-twitch" sports—baseball, football, basketball—that valued power over endurance. To some extent, this is still true.

Of course, there were always runners. At the turn of the twentieth century, the first Boston Marathons were run, and won, by blue-collar men: blacksmiths, carpenters, farmers, millers. Because of its annual showcase, Boston never lost its running culture. Meanwhile, around America—as well as in Britain, Japan, Finland, and Germany—small groups of committed men (and it was almost entirely men, at this stage, who competed at long distances) found a communion through running. But road racing was still not an accessible or attractive sport to the public at large.

Several moments helped alter this perception in America—

and then the world. In 1968, Dr. Kenneth Cooper published an influential and revolutionary book called *Aerobics,* which argued that regular aerobic exercise—be it running, cycling, or swimming—was good for you. Then, in 1972, Frank Shorter, a Yale graduate from an army family in upstate New York, won gold in the marathon at the Munich Olympics. He was the first American to do so since Johnny Hayes in 1908. But, unlike that famous race in London, Shorter's heroics in Munich were televised.

Marathons began to draw increasingly large fields. In the 1970s, a new sport called jogging became not only popular but oddly glamorous. Bill Bowerman started a little shoe company called Blue Ribbon Sports out of his garage in Oregon. The business later changed its name to Nike. Meanwhile, books like Jim Fixx's *The Complete Book of Running* sold hundreds of thousands of copies and spent weeks at the top of bestseller lists. Running was no longer just a sport for skinny beatniks; it was a sport for everyone. And the marathon, once seen as the most daunting of challenges, opened its arms.

———

The New York City Marathon was the catalyst for changing a popular sport into a professional one. Fred Lebow, who co founded the first New York City Marathon in 1970 and became its dominant impresario, was at the heart of this process. Born Ephraim Fischl Lebowitz in Arad, Romania, in 1932, Lebow survived the Holocaust and escaped Soviet Romania before living in Czechoslovakia, Ireland, and Kansas City. He finally settled in New York, where he worked in the textiles business in the Garment District of Manhattan.

Lebow was an ardent tennis player who competed in club

tournaments. One day in the 1960s, his doctor told him that the reason he lost big matches was his lack of stamina. So he started running. Pretty soon he had joined the New York Road Runners Club—a group of a few dozen men and women who raced around Yankee Stadium in the Bronx. Talking to the *New York Times* in 1980, he said that after he started running, he never lost another tennis match. "Of course," he added, "I haven't played one."

Like many subsequent converts to jogging, Lebow was an evangelist. But his enthusiasm didn't seem to rub off at first. The inaugural New York City Marathon in 1970 was short on glamour. Only 127 competitors started the course, which was a four-lap tour of Central Park. Lebow, who paid for safety pins and soft drinks out of his own pocket, placed 45th out of 55 finishers. There were fewer than a hundred spectators. The winner—in 2:31:39—was a firefighter named Gary Muhrcke, who had just completed a full night shift. He received a wristwatch for his efforts.

Six years later, a civil servant named George Spitz suggested to Lebow that the city of New York should create a new kind of marathon to honor the nation's bicentennial. Rather than run the race around Central Park—which was then a dingy criminal hot spot—Spitz suggested it should travel through all five boroughs. Lebow was skeptical at first, believing correctly that organizing such an event would be a knotty exercise in logistics. But having warmed up to the idea, he cajoled and coaxed services from desk jockeys throughout the boroughs. Soon New York City had a marathon worthy of its status.

The course for the five-borough race has been roughly the same ever since. The marathon begins in Staten Island, before the

Verrazano-Narrows Bridge, and passes through Brooklyn and Queens before hitting Manhattan at 16 miles. After going north on First Avenue, the athletes run a mile in the Bronx before swinging back into Manhattan on the Madison Avenue Bridge. The race then careens down Fifth Avenue and finishes in Central Park, next to the Tavern on the Green.

Lebow had a course. But if he was going to make the first five-borough marathon more than a scenic fun run, he needed stars. That meant he needed Frank Shorter and Bill Rodgers. Shorter was the 1972 Olympic champion and 1976 silver medalist in the marathon; Rodgers had broken the American record when winning the Boston Marathon in 1975. Lebow approached both men and they both agreed to race. There was a catch, however. Rodgers wanted money.

Lebow initially balked at the demand. For one thing, it flouted the rules of amateurism. But there was a greater principle at stake. As Cameron Stracher, author of an excellent account of the American running boom, *Kings of the Road*, suggests, "Lebow expected the athletes to donate their time in service to the greater good."

Rodgers saw it otherwise. Although he was a teacher by trade, he had dedicated large parts of his adult life to running. The previous year, he had been rated the number-one marathoner in the world. (He'd also been paid $1,000 to appear at the Enschede Marathon in Holland.) He needed to earn a little money from his talent, rules or no rules. Eventually, Lebow crumbled. Rodgers got his $3,000, and Lebow got his race. Shorter, meanwhile, remembers being paid $4,000.

On race day, Rodgers made good on his pay packet and won in 2:10:10 amid joyful, chaotic scenes in Central Park. The marathon was a knockout, garnering enthusiastic reports in the press and goodwill among officials. Since 1976, more than a million people have competed in the New York City Marathon. By its own estimation, the race now generates $340 million in revenue for the city each year.

That 1976 race became the template not only for future New York City Marathons but for city marathons in general. In the years to come, as Rodgers won title after title, marathon organizers from overseas came to borrow a little New York magic. For instance, the Berlin Marathon, once a pleasant but unremarkable jaunt through the Grunewald forest, was redirected through the streets of West Berlin in 1981, making it part of the city for a day. After the Berlin Wall came down in 1989, the race was rerouted again so that it passed through the old East and West Berlin. In that first true city-wide race, on September 30, 1990, three days before Germany was officially reunified, many runners wept as they passed underneath the Brandenburg Gate.

The biggest impact of Lebow's race would be in London. In 1979, Chris Brasher, the cofounder of the London Marathon, had run in New York. He was overwhelmed by the experience. In an article in the *Observer* newspaper, he wrote: "To believe this story, you must believe that the human race can be one joyous family, working together, laughing together, achieving the impossible. . . . Last Sunday, in one of the most trouble-stricken cities in the world, 11,532 men and women from 40 countries in the world, assisted by over a million black, white and yellow people, laughed and cheered and suffered during the greatest folk festival the world has seen. I wonder whether London could stage such a festival? We have the course, a magnificent course . . . but do we have the heart and hospitality to welcome the world?"

The answer was yes. The inaugural London Marathon, which was run in 1981, was an exuberant success. Its course owed much to New York—winding through some of the poorest parts of South East London right into the heart of the city. Since the first race, the event has snowballed. In 2014, 125,000 people applied in less than twelve hours for just over 10,000 ballot places.

As these "folk festivals" sprang up in major cities all over the world, the fastest marathon runners began to become bolder in their demands. It took some brave athletes to start that ball rolling. Looking back, Rodgers says he was hurt by the backlash against his standoff with the "shamateurism" that prevailed in his sport. "It was very frustrating," he remembers. "People would say, 'Runners aren't *athletes*, marathoners aren't *athletes*. . . .' I'd always felt this sport was a great sport, and very undervalued. And I think that's since been proven to be true."

In 1973, the year after Frank Shorter had won gold in Munich in front of an audience of millions, he wanted to travel from Florida, where he was training, to run in the Boston Marathon. There was no prize money on offer, but Shorter asked if Boston would pay his travel expenses: a $100 student standby plane ticket. The race organizers refused and lost their athlete. Because of their tightfistedness, Shorter did not run a Boston Marathon until 1978.

At the end of the 1970s and the beginning of the 1980s, however, several controversial moments paved the way for a new era of professional marathon running. For some time, there had been a standoff between the national governing body of the sport, known as The Athletics Congress (or TAC), and some elite runners who had organized themselves into the Association of Road Running Athletes (or ARRA). TAC wanted to abide by amateur rules set out by the International Association of Athletics Federations, and was attempting to construct a plan—involving indirect payments to athletes—that would help them do so. ARRA had a simpler idea: let runners compete for money. And so did Jordache, a blue-jeans company, which sponsored one of the defining events in the development of the sport.

At the "Jordache Marathon," which took place in Atlantic City, New Jersey, in September 1980, a $50,000 purse went straight to the athletes. Thirty-one elite runners took part, despite warnings from TAC that anybody who participated in such a race would be barred from international competition. The race itself was sluggish and athletically undistinguished. But the two winners—Ron Nabers for the men (2:31:06) and Katie McDonald for the women (3:04:57)—took home $15,000 each. It's strange to imagine now, but the simple fact that the winners were paid directly struck many as revolutionary.

It took a while for the big-city marathons to follow suit. In fact, before they supported the Atlantic City race, Jordache had first approached Fred Lebow and the New York City Marathon, offering a $250,000 purse, but Lebow was trying to work things out with TAC at the time and declined. Of course, athletes were still being paid by Lebow. It was a question of how open one could be about it.

George Hirsch, the publisher of *New York* magazine, who cofounded the five-borough New York City Marathon with Lebow, remembers that one of the reasons why officials were so wary about revealing payments to top athletes was political, rather than ethical. In the beginning, the city offered its services for free. When Lebow revealed in a book in 1981 that the top runners had, in fact, been paid for years, it created a headache for Mayor Ed Koch. "His feeling was that if the athletes were getting paid, the city should get paid," remembers Hirsch. Eventually, that's what happened. In exchange for policing and other services, the city took a small amount of money from New York Road Runners. Today, that figure has ballooned. NYRR now pays the city around $4 million every year the race is run.

By the early 1980s, it was clear to those who knew the sport that amateurism was unsustainable. In 1981, for instance, another open money race called the Cascade Run-Off was endorsed by the ARRA, who demanded that its athletes be allowed to make money *and* be eligible for the Olympics. Whereas the Jordache race had been seen by many as an anomaly, best ignored—Lebow called it a "freakshow"—the Cascade Run-Off caused a squall of controversy.

The situation became ridiculous. If the authorities maintained their firm stance on the need for track athletes to stay amateur, many talented people weren't going to make the 1984 Olympics. Moreover, if races weren't going to pay athletes well, the shoe companies would. Regardless of the personal motivations of the athletes, America needed its best runners available to compete. The United States was already beginning to lose out to Soviet countries, who openly supported their elite athletes.

By many accounts, Frank Shorter was instrumental in steering a way around this seemingly intractable problem. A lawyer by trade, he found a loophole in the International Olympic Committee rulebook and set up a "trust fund" so that runners could be paid for running races. The trust fund was just a way of saving face. Shorter says now: "The IAAF was looking for a solution to the problem surrounding the obvious Eastern Bloc funding of their athletes. We gave them the solution. . . . I'm not sure anyone was even audited to assure compliance."

As the decade wore on it became increasingly acceptable to pay prize money. And, after Bill Rodgers and others had forged the way, it was Alberto Salazar who was the first distance runner to become seriously remunerated by the sport. Salazar was a good-looking and driven Cuban-American kid. His father, José, had fought alongside Fidel Castro in the Cuban Revolution, but left the island when it became clear that Castro was creating a godless republic. The Salazars fled to Miami in 1960, and moved to Wayland, Massachusetts, in 1968. During training runs, José used to shout at Alberto, "A Salazar never quits!"

Alberto's fortitude was his greatest quality as a runner. He trained with a kind of religious fervor and competed at the edge of good sense. More than once, he was hospitalized after completing a race. His desire brought dividends. Salazar won three consecutive New York City Marathons (one in a world record of 2:08:13 that was later voided because the course was remeasured and found to be 148 meters short). In 1982, he also won the famous "Duel in the Sun" against Dick Beardsley at the Boston Marathon—a win from which, he says, he never recovered.

In 1981, Salazar recruited an agent from IMG, who represented many of America's top athletes, and struck a deal with Nike, worth a base salary of $50,000. He would be paid many hundreds of thousands of dollars more if he was successful at various races. At the time, this was more money than any distance runner had earned from a shoe company.

——

As the marathon opened up, so did promoters' imaginations. In 1992, Lebow offered a prize of $1 million for the first man to break two hours in his home city. The offer was a stunt. The world record in 1992 was 2:06:50. To expect someone to shave nearly seven minutes from the world record was preposterous. To ask them to do so in New York—the slowest of the major marathons—was Lewis Carroll fantasy. Hirsch remembers taking Lebow aside after he announced the million-dollar prize and telling him he was crazy, because he had created a jackpot nobody could hope to claim.

"You know that and I know that," said Lebow. "But one million dollars makes a great headline, and the public won't take us seriously if this is just an amateur sport."

Lebow reaped his headlines, but some may have spoiled his breakfast. In *Runner's World*, Joe Henderson excoriated the promoter who had "cheapened the sport" with his vulgar play. "Would [Michael] Jordan be told 'here's your chance to earn a million dollars per game, but you must score 150 points to earn it'?" he asked. "Of course not. Jordan is paid, and paid extremely well, to do the improbable, not the impossible."

Henderson's anger was righteous, but Lebow was a scrappy entrepreneur and he understood a central truth about the marathon: it has always needed to shout louder than other events to get heard. The two-hour play was a gimmick, but so what? The sport needed gimmicks.

Lebow also understood that the effect of professionalism on the big-city marathons had done little to increase public interest in the elite races. All that had changed was that money went from being paid under the table to being paid over the table—and, to this day, the sums involved in such "over-the-table" payments are not disclosed to the public.

The major effect of professionalism, meanwhile, was to widen the fields that arrived at marathons—which meant, in a zero-sum game, that the chances of a homegrown winner like Bill Rodgers or Frank Shorter narrowed. Indeed, as the 1980s and 1990s drew on, the cash prizes available in the best races in America, Europe, and the Far East began to attract athletes from every corner of the globe. And professionalism's most significant contribution? To draw athletes from East Africa, who now rule the sport.

——

Africa had been coming for a while. The American marathoner Kenny Moore recalls a moment from the Mexico City Olympics of 1968 in which that dominance appeared to become manifest. Ten miles into the Olympic marathon, Moore was sticking close to the Ethiopian favorite, Abebe Bikila. No doubt the Ethiopian was the man to watch. A soldier in Haile Selassie's Imperial Guard, he had become the first black African to win an Olympic gold, at the Rome Olympics in 1960, when he won the marathon in bare feet. Four years later, at the Tokyo Olympics, he repeated his heroics, this time in shoes.

But in the thin air of Mexico, Bikila was carrying an injury—and, 10 miles into the race, he decided to quit. Just before Bikila did so, he beckoned his fellow Ethiopian competitor, Mamo Wolde, toward him. Moore remembers the two men having a short conversation in Amharic. Many years later, having embarked on a successful career as a journalist for *Sports Illustrated*, Moore discovered what had been said between the two men:

"Lieutenant Wolde."

"Captain Bikila."

"I am not finishing this race."

"Sorry, sir."

"But Lieutenant, you will win this race."

"Sir, yes, sir."

"Don't let me down."

Wolde was as good as his word, and Ethiopia won its third marathon gold in succession.

You will win this race. Bikila gave it as an order. But today, it could just as easily be understood as a statement of fact. Athletes from East Africa have dominated distance running since at least the 1980s. That grip has only intensified, particularly in the marathon, and particularly in the past few years. All fifteen major marathons raced between the spring of 2011 and the fall of 2013 were won either by Kenyans or Ethiopians. Kenyans have won twelve; Ethiopians, three. From this group of major winners are men—rare, intriguing men—attempting to break new ground

Chapter Five

Anything Is Possible, Everything Is Possible

2008–2010

AFTER HIS first professional triumph in Monaco, Geoffrey Mutai returned from the land of pampered dogs to Kenya, the Rift Valley, and to Skyland. Everything and nothing had changed for him. In Kapng'tuny, his training mates slapped him on the back and told him well done. They asked for his stories from *outside*. And then everybody went back to work.

They gathered for the first run of each day before dawn, when the sky was still black and buckshot with stars. The men emerged from their shacks and cottages: fifty or sixty in hats and gloves and thin running jackets, holding themselves against the cold, shaking the hands of the other athletes as they arrived. When all had gathered at the hand-painted sign for the Kapng'tuny High School (motto: "Strive for Zenith"), the group set off into the high, dusty lanes.

Often, the first run of the day was an "easy ten"—10 kilometers at a canter; a wake-up call. But although these sessions were convivial, a product of running in a group in which nobody was attempting to press the accelerator, there was a seriousness to the endeavor. The athletes feared injury. If they were hurt, they could not train; if they could not train, they could not compete; if they did not compete, they could not earn money. There is no union, or sick pay, in road running.

The danger of working in the early morning on rough roads was considerable. The men mitigated this risk by arranging themselves into single files, each following a smooth tire track in the amber dust. When a rock or pothole was sighted, the foremost athlete would veer and point his arm straight down to indicate the threat. This signal was then passed backward to the runners behind. The effect was strangely moving to witness. Wordlessly, the runners became a platoon on a night exercise, an army on the move.

A few minutes into the workout, the sun would come up with equatorial swiftness—like a bounced tennis ball—causing the fields to glow a vivid fern green. Grazing cows observed the runners with doleful eyes. Farmers stopped to wave. There were few if any vehicles on the dirt roads. At a certain point in the run, the athletes would pass a train station named Ainabkoi, which hadn't seen a paying passenger since the late 1990s.

It was done in forty minutes. Having finished the run, the athletes arranged themselves once more around the high school sign, with sunlight on their backs and sweat on their brows. Stretching out their hamstrings on a grassy verge, they laughed, swapped jokes, and talked about the day ahead. Mutai returned to his cottage, drew water from a well, washed himself from the bucket, drank a cup or two of sweet tea, ate a piece of bread, and readied himself for the next session at 9 a.m.

——

As Mutai went back to work after Monaco—125 miles a week, more or less; uphill, downhill, fast and slow—so did his manager. Now that Mutai was a marathon winner, it was easier for Van de Veen to book him into other races. So Mutai took more planes, saw more crazy *muzungus*, smoked more rivals. In July, he won a flat 10km race in Voorthuizen, Holland, in a course record of 28:05. Then, in the fall, he won the Eindhoven Marathon—a second-tier European marathon that attracts a strong field—in a course record of 2:07:50.

The victory in Eindhoven came as a surprise even to Mutai. Eindhoven is known as a fast course, and he had gone there looking only to improve his personal best. He remembers consciously holding back his pace in the first half of the race, on the advice of his manager, and letting a group of more senior athletes go ahead of him. By halfway, however, Mutai was feeling so good that he quickened his pace to reel the leaders in. He caught them with ease and eventually left all his rivals in his wake—winning the race a minute and a half ahead of the next competitor. At the finish line, he experienced a minor epiphany. He now understood that he was not just another Kenyan runner. He knew then, in his own words, "I am talented."

When Mutai recognized his gift after that race in Eindhoven, it was as if he had put on a featherweight suit of armor. His confidence rose over the races and years to come. It was not arrogance, exactly. Given the way he lived, cheek by jowl with his training mates in the most rudimentary surroundings, he could never feel anything but an intense fellowship with other athletes. But he also knew he was different from most other runners. As his career developed, he would keep telling himself: *Anything is possible. Everything is possible.*

——

Mutai's commercial prospects also changed with the win in Eindhoven. By the end of 2008, he was a two-oh-seven guy, and that label came with its own bartering power.

The professional marathon is a strange sport in many respects. In the absence of global stars, television money has ebbed away from all but a few well-known races. The very best runners, however, continue to be paid well—and not just by their shoe company sponsors. The races themselves spend serious money for the fastest men. Oddly, this flow of cash to the elite fields is generated by the runners who finish far behind them. Not only do the hordes at the back of the field spend money to enter marathons—either personally or through charities—but, more important, they are rich pickings for advertisers. Amateur running is an activity for affluent people. In 2013, the American readers of *Runner's World* had an average household income of $106,963, much higher than many of the money magazines like *Forbes,* whose average was $85,955, or *Fortune,* whose average was $91,574. No wonder big-name sponsors such as Bank of America (for Chicago), ING and TCS (for New York City), and Virgin Money (for London) have spent their millions on the marathon.

This sponsors' cash pile is then reinvested in a few professionals who are paid to appear, to run fast, and to win. Even a small cash prize can dramatically improve the life of an East African runner. For instance, the $15,000 for first place in a regional Chinese marathon is enough to buy a significant plot of land back home.

In the second decade of the twenty-first century, the professional marathon scene is dominated by a few big races where appearance fees alone run to hundreds of thousands of dollars per athlete. These are the World Marathon Majors in New York, Boston, Berlin, Chicago, Tokyo, and London, which are arranged into a points system that awards the best male and female runner in a two-year period a half-million-dollar jackpot. There are also a host of second-tier events in places like Rotterdam, Seoul, Frankfurt, Paris, and Eindhoven, which offer substantial rewards, financial and reputational. All these events form an unofficial marathon "circuit," but they are essentially separate and competing fiefdoms.

Every professional runner obsesses about *time*. Fast times mean you become attractive to race organizers, which means you are invited to better events, which means more appearance money. In the Nandi Hills of Kenya, or on the training trails of Addis Ababa, athletes know each other not just by name but by personal best. That guy is a two-oh-eight. This one is a two-oh-five.

While each marathon is the standard distance, each city has its own quirks, and each race day its own personality. Aside from the weather, which is a potent factor in the marathon, there are a handful of other variables to take into consideration. Some courses are flat and some are hilly. Perhaps more significantly, some races employ pacemakers and some don't. Pacemakers not only help an elite runner hit his intended split times, but they also can shield him from the headwind that is generated—whatever the weather—by his own forward movement. (A wind tunnel study showed that if an athlete was protected from the wind by a rabbit over a whole marathon, while running at two-hour-marathon pace, he could save 100 seconds.)

Adding to this confusing picture is the composition of the elite field. It is a counterintuitive truth about the marathon that the stronger the field at an elite marathon the less likely it is that a course record will be set. With a few exceptions, records tend to be broken when the pace is fast and steady and dominated by one or two athletes. With too many studs testing each other's strength, the pace tends to rise and dip—breaking the athletes' rhythm and flooding their legs with lactic acid in the final stages—and the potential for fast times dissipates.

For all these reasons, one is never comparing like with like. However, some marathons are attractive because they are known to be fast. First among them is Berlin, which has held the men's world record for the past decade and books star runners who come to the German capital with the express goal of lowering the mark. But on the right day, Frankfurt, Dubai, or Rotterdam could be Berlin's equal. Athletes will often choose to run a "fast" marathon, where they may be paid less, in order to run a new personal best, and then parlay their new status as a two-oh-four guy into an invitation to race at one of the big paydays like New York or London.

This was the game in which Mutai was now engaged. Of course, he wanted to win marathons, but he also needed to sharpen his personal best in order to progress to better marathons. The ultimate goal was to race and win at the Majors. If he was to make good on the wellspring of talent he knew was within his own body, he would need not only to maintain his devotion to training, but to plot a canny path between races.

In 2009, that meant traveling to Daegu, in South Korea, where—struggling with an injury—he limped to an eighth-place finish. Then, healed and revived by an uninterrupted block of training, he returned to the Voorthuizen 10km, where he shattered his own course record in 27:39. Next he went back to the Eindhoven Marathon, where he ran a measured opening 35km in windy conditions, before running the fastest closing stretch in the history of the sport. It was a dazzling move that shattered the field. Mutai covered the final 7.195 kilometers at Eindhoven in 20 minutes, 28 seconds at 2:50 per km—or, in layman's terms, exactly two-hour-marathon pace. Van de Veen, who was following on a motorcycle, says he almost literally could not believe his eyes. It was as if a switch had been flicked in his athlete. Mutai remembers a profound joy in those final kilometers. This was the Spirit. He felt it most when running alone, at the front of a broken field, faster and faster.

Mutai won the race in another new course record of 2:07:01. At the postrace press conference, a journalist asked whether his victory was ever in doubt. No, he said, without braggadocio. It was just a fact. He was, he knew, the strongest athlete in the field. What's more, he said, "I know I can be faster than this."

Six weeks later, at the Valencia half marathon—way too soon, you would think, for another great performance—Mutai held off the challenge of an outstanding field that included his friend and future two-oh-three guy Wilson Kipsang to win the race in 59:30. The weather was too hot and too windy for those kinds of times, but Mutai somehow prevailed in what was then the fastest half-marathon debut in history. He burned with confidence. At every startline, he felt ready, in his own words, to let his "body talk."

"People who I feared, that fear went away," he remembers.

——

This spirit of ambition had infected the sport. The simple fact of being a Kenyan marathoner runner was emboldening. Almost all lucrative marathons in this period were won by Kenyans and Ethiopians—and, out of those two countries, Kenya took the lion's share. Nations who had once provided winners—countries like Britain, New Zealand, the United States, Japan—had faded from the reckoning.

But even in this generally encouraging environment, there was something singular in the air at the time Mutai emerged as a professional marathoner: a fissile atmosphere in which boundary breaking became the norm. Two athletes in particular—one a doyen, nearing the end of his peak, and one a young novice, tragically nearing the end of his life—changed the way the world thought about racing.

First the old man. Haile Gebrselassie, who is known universally by his first name, was born into a large family in the thin air of Arsella, Ethiopia, sometime in the early to mid-1970s. His official birth date is April 18, 1973, but nobody, not even Haile, seems to know exactly when he was born. His parents worked the land and expected their son one day to do the same. But Haile was raised on tales of Ethiopia's marathon heroes of the 1960s, Abebe Bikila and Mamo Wolde, and wished only to run. As a boy, he ran six miles to school and back every weekday to avoid a beating from his teacher, or his violent, disciplinarian father—whoever he was late for. He built a career on these youthful exertions. Throughout his time as a professional runner, Haile never ironed out a kink in his technique—a crook in his left elbow where he had once carried his schoolbooks.

Haile is now widely considered to be the greatest distance runner of all time. His best years came on the track. Among other honors, he won four world championship gold medals and two Olympic golds at 10,000m—both the product of thrilling duels with his Kenyan archrival Paul Tergat. (It was the second of these gold medals that lionized Haile in the eyes of Geoffrey Mutai, who was watching on a barroom television and breaking out in sweats.) Later in his career, he switched to the roads, where he picked his races carefully, broke two marathon world records in Berlin, and ensured a profound legacy. Garrulous, smart, and handsome, he remains the sport's only true African star—a fact that continues to trouble race organizers, sponsors, and television executives.

His reputation in the marathon, however, is a complicated one. Despite the fact that Haile broke the marathon world record twice, few aficionados would call him the greatest marathoner of all time. Along with his rival Tergat, he came to road racing in the latter stages of his peak—in his late twenties or early thirties, depending on your interpretation of his age—and sometimes faltered at the marathon distance when challenged by a serious opponent in prime condition. Mutai, for whom Haile will always be a hero, says that the Ethiopian could not perform when other runners "looked at his legs"—that is, when he was crowded in.

But there is no doubting Haile's physical gifts. Some scientists believe that if Haile had come to the marathon earlier, the two-hour marathon might already be broken. In 2011, three exercise physiologists from the faculty of medicine at Aix-Marseille University in France made this case in the *Journal of Applied Physiology*. The French team used a model showing that the VO_2 max, or maximal oxygen uptake, of the athlete who breaks two hours must measure 86 ml.kg.-1.min.-1 (you don't need to know anything about these numbers, except that they are extraordinary). Then the scientists argued that aging lowers VO_2 max linearly by 0.43 ml/kg/min every year. Given that Gebrselassie's VO_2 max reading at the time of breaking the marathon world record in Berlin in 2008 was 82.8, they estimated that he would have been able to break the two-hour barrier in the year 2000, just about the time he was winning his last Olympic gold medal in the duel with Paul Tergat. "Thus," they wrote, "we predict that a world class marathon runner from East Africa, aged around 25 years or less, could break the 2h barrier if specifically trained early enough."

The Aix-Marseille theory is interesting, but it leads one down a blind alley as far as Haile is concerned. For one thing, runners are much more than their VO_2 max. More important, Haile didn't run his first marathon until 2002, and he has never believed in running marathons young. "It's the bone, the joint," he told me. "It's very soft. . . . If you cut a young tree for timber, you cannot succeed. The wood is very soft, the strength is poor. Because it's young. The same thing for the human being."

Haile may not have been at his fastest when he came to the marathon, but he was strong as an oak and world famous. He knew where his talents lay, and he adapted. Most of his wins came in races in Berlin and Dubai: fast courses, arranged for his pleasure. He never won a tactical race in New York or London, against deep, strong fields. In fact, Haile made it an explicit condition of his appearance in some marathons that certain rivals not be invited.

What Haile did for the marathon, however, was to change the way the sport thought about world records. Before Haile, world records were broken as a result of *racing*. The time itself was not the goal, but rather a bonus—a happy by-product. If a world record fell, great. If it was missed, nobody cried. The idea of setting up a race with pacers for the convenience of one or two strong athletes with world record intentions was an alien one.

At Haile's first marathon, in London in 2002, the world record was broken in a sensational three-way tussle that saw the Ethiopian reeled in by Tergat and the eventual winner, Khalid Khannouchi, a Moroccan-born American. For many in the sport, London 2002 was the greatest race they had seen. It had everything: speed, personality, drama, and—it was almost an afterthought—a world record.

In some ways, that race in London was a watershed. Later in the decade, Haile began to use his star power to negotiate his appearance at marathons—at Berlin, in particular—where the express purpose was to break a world record. He didn't want a race but a time, and the marathon organizers commandeered the services of some outstanding athletes to keep pace for him.

Haile wasn't the first to think of this strategy. Berlin has always been attractively flat and fast. In 2003, Tergat raced in Berlin with pacemakers and world record intentions. The marathon was not as well ordered as he might have liked; unusually, he ended up in a battle with one of his own rabbits, Sammy Korir. But the result was exceptional. Tergat won the race and became the first man in history to break 2:05.

Haile took this nascent template and adjusted it to his own purposes. With his manager, Jos Hermens, he also developed a more scientific approach. In Tergat's record-beating year, the leading athletes ran a relatively slow first half and quickened in the second. Haile knew this was an inefficient use of energy, and that simply by organizing a more evenly paced race, he could take seconds out of Tergat's time.

With the help of Sean Hartnett, a cartographer from the University of Wisconsin and a running journalist, Haile had maps drawn up of the Berlin course with targeted split times written on them. He stuck images of the Berlin route all around his gym, and in his office, so that he could memorize the course and his intended split times in his head. On marathon day, said Hartnett, Haile hoped "to race the times" rather than his competitors.

Perhaps the more important development was a technological one. With Hartnett's help, Haile became the first athlete at a major marathon to benefit from live split times on an electronic display from the race vehicle. He could see, in real time, what time he had run in total, and for the last kilometer. He could also see a projected finishing time on the screen. This display was dubbed "the Haile Board."

Twice at Berlin, in 2007 and 2008, these strategies paid off. In 2007, Haile broke Tergat's record in 2:04:26. The next year, with refined pacing strategy and an even more detailed live display, he broke it again, in 2:03:59. It wasn't only the technology that made Haile run fast. But what he understood, perhaps better than anyone, is how planning a race was the key to records. (In the 1920s and 1930s, "the Flying Finn" Paavo Nurmi was the first famous runner to discuss this philosophy of measured pacing. It served him well: he broke 22 world records in his career.)

Establishing open world record attempts in the marathon was only a development of what had long been a feature of track athletics. Ever since the quest to crack the four-minute mile in the 1950s, races had periodically been arranged with the express purpose of record breaking. Roger Bannister's own breakthrough sub-four-minute mile in Oxford, in 1954, was set up beautifully by two fellow athletes—including Chris Brasher, later a cofounder of the London Marathon—who brought their lanky friend through three-quarters of a mile in perfect time.

But Haile was the first man to openly employ Bannister's time-trial idea in the marathon. It was a galvanizing moment for the sport. Haile understood that records were broken by athletes who prepared to break records. And they were broken "in the mind" before they were broken with the feet. To thrust yourself to the limits of your running capacity for two hours, said Haile, required a special kind of personality. Anyone attempting to run so fast knew that there was a strong chance his body might buckle under the strain, and that he might not only lose the race, but fail to complete it. That kind of implosion came with all kinds of penalties: to your career, to your confidence, and to your bank balance. Pioneers, said Haile, had to be brave.

——

Sammy Wanjiru was a different kind of brave than Haile, but he changed the sport just as radically. A short, powerful Kikuyu from Kenya's Central Province, he blazed through the marathon world before his death at the age of twenty-four in 2011.

The race for which Wanjiru is best known came on the final day of the 2008 Beijing Olympics. Before 2008, surprisingly, no Kenyan had ever won the Olympic marathon—a fact some Kenyans attributed to the lack of prize money. The conditions in Beijing were set to be oppressive, with heat, humidity, and pollution all thickening the air. Haile was so concerned about the weather

and the smog that he pulled out of the Olympics some weeks before the race. (He chose, instead, to race in Berlin that fall, where
he broke the world record.) For the remaining competitors, the
sensible thing to do in the circumstances would have been to run
an easy pace and challenge for the lead in the closing stages of
the marathon.

Sammy had little time for wisdom of any kind. He was twenty-
one years old, in the shape of his life, and he felt bulletproof. He
decided to torch a rapid pace from the first mile and see who
could follow. The answer was nobody. Some months after the
race, Wanjiru described his tactics to a Spanish journalist. "It's
easy to explain," he said. "I pushed hard from the gun and whenever I realized that one athlete was able to live with my pace I
made another kick to leave him behind."

When Sammy reached the Bird's Nest stadium in first place,
there was no one around him. He could have coasted to the finish
line. Instead, he sprinted the last few hundred yards, saluting the
roaring crowd on each side. His time was 2:06:32, which broke
the Olympic record by almost three minutes. Having watched
Sammy's performance, Dave Bedford, the organizer of the London Marathon, said that Wanjiru had become "instantly the best
and most exciting marathon runner in the world, maybe ever. . . .
The conditions called for a slow, tactical race. Nobody was ex-
pecting a front-running onslaught."

Bedford was not the only startled observer. In the Olympic
race, Sammy changed how people thought of the marathon. After
2008, it was no longer seen as a pure endurance event in which
athletes hung on until the closing miles to make their move. In
Beijing, Sammy had shown that the distance didn't frighten him.
He simply motored away, mile after mile, and dared others to

join him. The fact that he won in such a manner sent a powerful message to elite runners everywhere: speed kills.

Sammy was also different from most other East African runners in that he made no secret of his talent, or his ambitions. In early 2009, a few months after the Olympics, he told a reporter that he intended to break two hours for the marathon within the next five years. Tragically, he did not live long enough to be proved wrong.

——

Sammy's childhood was tough. He grew up in a mud hut in a small village called Githunguri, which sat on a hill in the heart of Kikuyu country near the market town of Nyahururu. He didn't know his real father—although several men later claimed that honor—and his mother often went away for long periods to look for work. As a kid, Sammy was often cared for by his grandparents.

Because of the family's arable plot, there was enough to eat but rarely enough money to do much but survive. He left school at twelve because there were no funds for school fees. And, like many top Kenyan runners, he did not own a pair of shoes until he was a teenager. Still, he trained regularly at the Nyahururu Municipal Stadium, a run-down dirt track with an overgrown soccer field in its center.

The turning point in Sammy's life came at around fifteen years of age, when he was spotted by a Japanese agent. For twenty years or so, there had been a tradition of Kikuyu runners traveling to Japan to compete in *ekiden*—popular, and often televised, long-distance relays. When Sammy was asked if he would like to go to Japan to finish his schooling on a running scholarship, he leapt at the opportunity. He also admitted that he had no idea where Japan was.

Away from home, Sammy thrived on the track and the roads. He trained hard, broke records, and earned the admiration of his Japanese peers. But his social life was difficult. There was a new language to learn and new customs to internalize. For a testosterone-flooded teenager, it was hard to live a normal life. Kenyans who have trained in Japan say it is almost impossible for an African man to find a Japanese girlfriend. His former coach also believes Sammy developed a taste for alcohol there.

Wanjiru graduated from high school in 2005 and joined the Toyota Kyushu running team under the tutelage of the 1992 marathon silver medalist, Koichi Morishita. He soon began to make a mark on the world stage. Six months after graduating, he smashed the world junior record for the 10,000m in 26:41.75. Two weeks later, he broke Paul Tergat's world half-marathon record in Rotterdam with a time of 59:16. (Sammy lost the half-marathon record in 2006 to Zersenay Tadese and then to Haile. He recaptured it in 2007, in 58:53, then lowered it again, to 58:33. It now belongs to Tadese, at 58:23.)

Many talented young distance runners struggle when they step up to the marathon. Sammy made the distance look like a breeze. At his debut, in Fukuoka in December 2007, he won in 2:06:39—a course record and, at the time, the second-fastest debut ever run. He then finished second to the great Martin Lel in London before making himself world famous with his Olympic gold. By the time he was twenty-one, Sammy had signed a contract with Nike, was an Olympic champion, and had earned more than a million dollars from racing.

Wanjiru's real trouble was at home. In 2005, long before he was famous, he met and married a girl from Nyahururu named Terezah Njeri. ("Married" can be a loose term in Kenya. A man who lives with another woman is said to be married to her.) Njeri's relationship with Wanjiru's mother, Hannah, would be a continuous source of heartache for the rest of his life.

I met Njeri shortly after Wanjiru died, at the bar next to a roaring waterfall where her husband would often drink into the night with his pals. She had a gorgeous, doll-like face, a tiny voice, and six fingers on her right hand. Njeri said she couldn't have married Wanjiru for his money. When they first became a couple, he didn't have any. "It was me who earned the money back then," she said. "I had a job at the salon. When he stayed in town, we all lived together—me, Sammy, and his mother—in the same room."

This claustrophobic arrangement sparked a long-standing enmity between the two most significant women in the runner's life. Njeri said that Hannah Wanjiru "always hated me." Luckily for Sammy, in the months that followed his marriage, he was often away. But when he sent money home, his wife and mother quarreled. At the heart of the dispute was the question of control. Njeri says that "Sammy could not buy a present for me without his mother getting jealous."

In 2006 and 2007, Wanjiru built two large, ugly houses in Nyahururu—one for him and his wife, and one for his mother. They were only fifty yards apart and created rival power bases. A few years later, having married another woman in a traditional ceremony, he established his new wife in a house *between* his mother's and his own.

Wanjiru also had a problem with money. He burned it, and it burned him. In a pattern that continued for the rest of his life, he sent mountains of cash back to Nyahururu, bought cars at several times their proper value, and entered into business relationships and property deals where his supposed partners robbed him blind. After his death, Wanjiru's lawyer, Ndegwa Wahome, told *Sports Illustrated* that his client was seen as the softest of touches. For an apartment complex Wanjiru was building in nearby Nakuru, he "probably spent 10 times the cost." Wahome added: "Some of the people working there took so much of the materials that they built their own houses."

Sammy also had an appetite for alcohol that was unleashed particularly at times of high stress. He was not the first or last Kenyan runner to suffer with drink. Rural Kenya, in particular, is in the grip of an alcoholism epidemic. Part of the problem is the binary view Kenyans have formed about drink. One is either a "drunkard" or one is not. The idea of having one or two beers, or a glass of wine with dinner, makes no sense. In the countryside, the majority of the men who drink do so to extreme. Sammy was not a drunkard in the traditional sense, because he could control his appetites during times of hard training. But once he had a taste, he was on a one-way street.

Sammy's lifestyle took a while to exact its penalty. He still clocked superb performances. In 2009, he won both the London and Chicago marathons in course records. The Chicago time of 2:05:41 was the fastest ever recorded on American soil. These two runs helped him win the World Marathon Majors jackpot of $500,000 and gave him the confidence to claim that Gebrselassie's world record was in his sights. But it was obvious to anyone who saw his domestic situation in the years following the Olympics that his behavior was not suited to that of a champion.

"He started to change after Beijing," says Njeri. "He got new friends—some good, some bad. He started to take alcohol. He refused to go to training sometimes. When he was with me, he was so good. He loved his kids. He couldn't go to sleep without knowing they were okay. But when he was with his friends, I don't know what happened to him."

There were so many claims on Sammy's attention. At the time of his death, there were three women who called themselves his wife, as well as several girlfriends. It was not just his lovers who wanted something from him. He was never alone. Eighteen hours a day, someone—a girlfriend, a cousin, a stranger—demanded his attention, or his wallet. He built houses for his wives and relatives, rented houses for girlfriends, covered his friends' restaurant bills, and paid for less successful athletes' shoes and travel. Wanjiru's friends told me he was paying dozens of children's school fees. Months after his death, there was still a bare patch of earth outside the front gate of his house where people waited for Sammy the Munificent to emerge and dispense his plentiful baksheesh. Claudio Berardelli, his former coach—an impassioned Italian in his early thirties with a shaved head and the physique of the racing cyclist he once was—remembers: "Sammy's great problem is that he could never say no."

It was only in 2010 that Sammy's life began to unravel in public. When he failed to complete the 2010 London Marathon, his Italian manager, Federico Rosa, decided to intervene. Rosa and Berardelli took Sammy to Italy for a liver toxicity test. The results showed that he had not yet created lasting damage from his drinking, but Berardelli told Rosa to "scare" Sammy with the results in order to encourage him to live clean. After the London disappointment, Berardelli was also assigned to monitor Sammy more closely.

Berardelli liked Wanjiru, and respected his awesome abilities. Together with Rosa, he attempted to rescue him. In July 2010, the coach invited Sammy to attend a camp in Italy with other athletes. The world's best marathon runner was overweight, out of shape, and could not stay with his training partners on a fifty-minute run. Then, in August, Berardelli invited Sammy to stay with him in his house in Eldoret, far away from the temptations and crushing atmosphere of his hometown.

According to Berardelli, Wanjiru was happier in Eldoret. He stopped drinking and was training regularly. But he was still in bad shape. Two weeks before he was due to defend his title at the Chicago Marathon, Berardelli was convinced that he should pull Sammy out of the race. But the runner kept saying to his coach, "Let me try, let me try." Berardelli traveled to the Windy City with no great hope.

The performance that Sammy produced in Chicago in 2010 was unexpected and unforgettable. Somehow, he summoned the willpower to resist a series of bold moves by Tsegaye Kebede, his rival for the $500,000 World Marathon Majors jackpot. In the final mile or so, the lead changed five times. Sammy messed with his rival's head—by running in his shadow, switching sides behind him, and by reacting to Kebede's feints with sprints of his own. Toni Reavis, commentating on the race from a motorcycle alongside Mike Adamle and Ed Eyestone for NBC, almost lost his voice in the excitement. Their call of the final mile or so of the Chicago race is a reminder of the zenith of recent professional marathoning.

"Here's Wanjiru now! Ha! Shoulder to shoulder . . . There goes Sammy hard. . . . Remember there's $500,000 on the line for the winner. . . . Wow! Sammy's been broken three times and he refuses to give in. . . . This is like Frazier Ali. . . . Kebede . . . He can't put a stake in his heart! Each time you think Kebede's broken Wanjiru, he just fights right back, he refuses to go gently. . . .

There goes Kebede again. . . . What a race . . . What can you say? Eight hundred yards to go . . . There he goes hard, hard, hard, hard. . . . This is unbelievable! Wanjiru thought he was going to come by him, but Kebede rallies and comes back. . . . The last little hill on the course . . . Now it's Wanjiru. . . . This is the first time Sammy's been in front! He might do it! Look at that guy! Look at Wanjiru! Oh my gosh . . . This is a knockout punch right here. . . . This race is over! What *balls* this guy's got! Unbelievable victory! This is the greatest race of his life. . . ."

Shortly before cresting the tape, Sammy pointed to the crowd on each side of the final stretch. He then pointed straight forward, as if in a salute. It was a piece of showmanship utterly in keeping with his bravura performance, and it broke Kebede. After the race, the little Ethiopian wept.

One evening in June 2013, Berardelli watched the video of that final mile of Chicago 2010 in his house in Eldoret. The coach had been in Chicago for the race, and had also seen the footage dozens of times. Nevertheless, it still gave him chills. When his pistoning athlete crested the tape in triumph, Berardelli appeared quiet and wistful. You could understand why. Seven months after that sunny morning on Columbus Drive, Sammy was dead. The footage showed the last time Wanjiru raced.

———

It's no coincidence that Wanjiru died so soon after a triumph. His finest and ugliest days were intimately connected. The rewards on offer to the best marathon runners in this period had the capacity to change lives and minds. His final Chicago Marathon alone provided a huge windfall. He received $500,000 for winning the Marathon Majors jackpot, $115,000 for the race win itself, a further $200,000–400,000 in appearance fees, and an undisclosed bonus from Nike. He had to pay U.S. taxes, and his management's cut, but it was still astonishing money for a guy who wore his first pair of shoes only ten years earlier.

Berardelli believes Sammy earned around $8 million in his career. In Nyahururu, a decent family income for one year might total 80,000 Kenyan shillings, or a little more than $900. The journey between where Sammy came from and where he arrived was dizzying.

In his final two years, as the money and the booze flowed, his life became increasingly fraught—particularly where women were involved. By Christmas 2010, his relationship with Njeri reached its nadir. On December 28, Njeri called the police alleging that Sammy had threatened to kill her with an AK-47 assault rifle. He was arrested and bailed. Njeri subsequently asked for a divorce, before reconciling with Wanjiru before television news cameras in a bizarre stunt on Valentine's Day 2011.

Njeri encouraged the police to drop the attempted murder charge but the charge of handling an illegal weapon could not be wished away. Wanjiru was due in court on May 25, 2011. In the meantime, Wanjiru decided to buy Njeri a house in the Ngong Hills, outside Nairobi, to move her away from his mother. But, in her place, he collected new girlfriends. The drinking intensified. In April 2011, Wanjiru's best friend, Daniel Gatheru, called Berardelli and Rosa to blow the whistle.

Berardelli remembered Gatheru telling him: "Please guys, get him out of here; it's the only solution. He is completely under pressure, and I have to pull him out every morning from the house to train. He's a little bit confused. He doesn't want to talk about his private problems."

Rosa and Berardelli told Wanjiru that he needed to sever ties with his life in Nyahururu. He was to stay at his coach's house in Eldoret, then travel to Oregon to train. Barring further mishap, he would target the New York City Marathon in November 2011 as his comeback. If he could steer his life back onto the road, there was no limit to what he might achieve; there were world records to assault and his Olympic gold medal to defend. Federico Rosa also says he believed in Wanjiru's boast: if anyone was capable of assaulting the two-hour marathon, it was Sammy.

———

In the week before his death, Wanjiru and Gatheru traveled to Eldoret and stayed with Berardelli. They slept early and trained hard. It was as happy as the Italian had ever seen his athlete. But only days before he was due to travel to America to continue training and escape his hometown worries, Sammy returned to Nyahururu to discuss the weapons charge with his lawyer.

On the drive home, Sammy got drunk everywhere from Nakuru to Nyahururu. At around 11 p.m., he arrived in the Kawa Falls Hotel in his hometown, where he met a girlfriend named Jane Nduta. According to Nduta, Wanjiru ordered two fried eggs, drank some wine, visited another bar, drove home, and passed out next to her. Soon, Terezah Njeri came back to the house and discovered him in bed with Nduta. An argument between the two women ensued. Njeri then padlocked the bedroom door, locking her unconscious husband and his girlfriend in the room together.

Although what happened next is still a matter of intense debate, it appears most likely that Wanjiru woke up and attempted to climb down from his bedroom balcony to continue the argument with Njeri. Clambering over the balustrade, he slipped, fell, landed on the back of his head, and died.

Not everyone believes this version of events, and Sammy's death is still the subject of conspiracy theories. Certainly the local police did nothing to dampen the gossip. At first, detectives said Sammy had committed suicide. Then they said it was an accident. Then a coroner leaked a preliminary postmortem report that suggested Sammy might have landed on all fours before being murdered by a blow to the back of the head. Years later, investigators in Kenya have never formally concluded their investigation or issued a definitive autopsy report. In the absence of concrete information, wild stories have flourished.

Berardelli believes that Wanjiru's death was an accident. When *Sports Illustrated* showed Wanjiru's postmortem report to Michael Baden, a U.S. pathologist, Baden said it showed a "typical contrecoup injury to the head" with a fracture at the back of the skull and bruising at the front of the head where the brain had slammed into the skull wall. The pathologist said that such an injury was consistent with a fall from ten feet, rather than being hit with a blunt object. In other words, Wanjiru's injuries appeared to be consistent with an accident rather than foul play.

Two months after the accident, Sammy had still not been buried. During a wide-ranging family squabble, Hannah Wanjiru refused to inter her son before his cause of death had been established. In one incident, captured on camera and posted to a national newspaper website, she attacked members of her own family with a machete as they inspected the burial site. Meanwhile, girlfriends and spurious relatives emerged seemingly daily from the woodwork, each with his or her own specious claim to Wanjiru's millions. They are still coming, years later.

Eventually, the funeral took place with a police guard. Sammy's mother did not attend. The body was taken to the Nyahururu athletics track before being buried in the back garden of Wanjiru's farm, ten minutes out of town. A pink marble headstone was erected, which bears the legend: IN LOVING MEMORY OF SAMUEL KAMAU WANJIRU. YOU FOUGHT THE GOOD FIGHT, FINISHED THE RACE, AND KEPT THE FAITH. YOU WILL LIVE FOREVER WITHIN OUR HEARTS.

Three days after the funeral, I visited the plot with Gatheru. A wheelbarrow filled with earth stood next to the grave. In the background, some thin Friesian cows—who would die of neglect months later—fed with their tails facing their old boss. For a few seconds, Gatheru stood with his head bowed and one of his bright blue Nike sneakers cocked against the headstone, in silence. The greatest marathon runner of his generation was dead at twenty-four, and his best friend could find nothing useful to say about it. But a hundred miles north, in the Kalenjin heartlands, Wanjiru's story was spoken like a parable.

Chapter Six

Kids, That Was Real

2010–2012

B Y 2010, Mutai knew he possessed rare talent. He also knew that talent was not enough. For the best runners, money swirled around and distractions were manifold. Every one of them had grown up like Sammy Wanjiru, poor and hungry. Mutai was not immune to such temptations. He remembered those foggy mornings in Rongai when he woke up in strangers' houses, and he understood how easy it would be to return to that life. Running country was full of squandered, drunken talent.

At the same time, he was excited by the ambition he saw around him. Athletes were achieving previously unthinkable times, and winning races in new ways. Haile had remade the art of record breaking in Berlin, and Wanjiru had reshaped the narrative of racing. One could not help but be swept up in the spirit of the age. Haile, in particular, inspired Mutai.

Every event became, in Mutai's words, "a graduation." Behind the scenes, his management was working to give him a shot at the Majors. After a lucrative sub-one-hour half-marathon win at Ras al-Khaimah in the United Arab Emirates, he was booked to run the Rotterdam Marathon in the spring of 2010. The race is not a Major, but it is in the highest class of second-tier marathons. Mostly people choose Rotterdam because, on the right day, it's fast.

On the gray, dank morning of April 11, 2010, the race started off rapidly. Ten contenders in the leading group sped through the first half in under 62 minutes, all of them on world record pace—a situation that could not hold. The lead group soon splintered and eventually included only two men: Mutai and Patrick Makau, a recalcitrant Kamba who wears a pencil mustache like a 1940s screen idol. In the closing straightaway, Makau pulled ahead of Mutai to record what was then the fourth-fastest marathon time ever: 2:04:47. Mutai was eight seconds behind, with a massive new personal best of 2:04:55. Although he hadn't won the race, he'd led Makau most of the way to the finish line. What's more, he was now a two-oh-four guy.

On the strength of his Rotterdam performance, Mutai was invited for a rematch against Makau in Berlin in September— his first Major. It was a rainy day, with puddles on the ground. Nobody expected a record. Once again, Mutai tried to push the pace; once again, Makau stuck to his heels. The pair ran as if linked by a tow chain all the way to the Brandenburg Gate, about 400 meters from the finish line, where Makau once again used his superior sprint to best his rival. The two men finished in 2:05:08 and 2:05:10, respectively.

This second consecutive defeat to Makau prompted a period of soul-searching for Mutai. He tried to analyze what had gone wrong. On both occasions, he had felt strong both before and during the race. He knew he was capable of *sustained* attacks of speed, as he had shown most dramatically at the 2009 Eindhoven Marathon, when he closed the last 7km in two-hour-marathon pace. But in Berlin and Rotterdam he had not burned off Makau with a sustained attack. Instead, he had merely escorted a faster finisher to the closing stages of the race like the world's best pacemaker, and then had politely watched him sprint past him. "What was embarrassing for me was, when I finished with Makau, I was still having energy," he remembered. "Why was I waiting? If I fight for it at the beginning, I would leave him. . . . That was the lesson that Makau teaches me."

To put the lesson another way: he needed to be more aggressive. He needed—his word—"courage." Most marathoners hate to front run. It's lonely. You are unprotected from the wind. It's psychologically tiring. You give the athletes behind you something to shoot at. In the past, however, there have been some special athletes who took strength from front running. Ron Clarke, the great Australian of the 1960s, was one of them.

For Clarke, front running was not just a tactic but an extension of his worldview. "The single most horrible thing that can happen to a runner is to be beaten in the stretch when he's still fresh," he told *Sports Illustrated*. "No matter who I was racing or what the circumstances, I tried to force myself to the limit over the whole distance. It makes me sick to see a superior runner wait behind the field until 200 meters to go and then sprint away. That is immoral. It's both an insult to other runners and a denigration of his ability."

Steve Prefontaine, the tragically short-lived American runner of the 1970s, was another front-runner, but he was less high-minded in his rhetoric. "I hate to have people back there sucking on me," he said.

Mutai needed some of Clarke and Prefontaine's attitude. He needed to kill off the suckers early. With his new plan in mind, he started to train differently. Back at his training camp in Kapng'tuny, he approached his weekly long run like it was a race day, and tried out his new tactic—building a fast pace until halfway, and then scorching ahead of his training partners on his own, to see how much pain, and speed, he could sustain. The answer, it seemed, was plenty. In 2011, armed with his new approach to marathon running, he would change the sport forever.

———

Mutai had never visited the United States before he arrived at Logan International Airport for the 2011 Boston Marathon. He came on the Tuesday before the Monday race—a little earlier than elite runners normally arrive—excited about the prospect of running a marathon he had seen so many times on television. Almost the first thing he wanted to do when he landed was to drive the length of the course. With Van de Veen, he took a car from Hopkinton, Massachusetts, all the way along the marathon's east-northeast trajectory toward the finish line at Boylston Street in the city's downtown. From watching previous marathons, the race's landmarks were familiar to him: Wellesley, Newton, Heartbreak Hill. But seeing the route up close for the first time, he was thrilled and a little intimidated. There were hills, lots of them. The course reminded him of his Skyland training tracks. When he got back to the hotel, he sought out his friend and fellow Kipsigis, Robert Cheruiyot, who had broken the course record at Boston the previous year in 2:05:52. "How did you run two-oh-five on *this*?" Mutai asked him. They both laughed.

The race day broke bright, cool, and windy from the west. It was perfect. Mutai, emboldened by his training and fortified by his new mantras—*kill them early; anything is possible; be brave*—settled into the race quickly. But it was Ryan Hall, the American, who pushed the pace in the early stages. He led the race alone, ahead of a large group of Africans. Sometimes he cupped his hand to his ear to encourage the crowd into frenzied cheering.

It had been a long time since Bostonians had celebrated an American man at the head of the marathon. Mutai remembers his fellow East Africans in the pack were not concerned by a white American making a break; they were sure they would be able to reel him in later. The only thing they worried about was a Kenyan or Ethiopian moving away from them. But Mutai was determined not to let Hall out of his sights. He respected the *muzungu's* ability and worried about allowing him too large a lead.

The miles rattled along. Encouraged and often led by Hall, a large lead group of about a dozen sped through halfway in 61:58—a very fast split, a minute and a half faster than Cheruiyot's halfway mark from the previous year. When Mutai pressed, six men responded. He made another bold move with around 7 miles to go, running a 4:32 mile between miles 19 and 20: under two-hour-marathon pace. Most of the pack, including Hall, crumbled under this assault. One man, a debutant named Moses Mosop, did not.

Mosop ran with a graceful, powerful action. As a junior, he was nicknamed Engine Kubwa—"Big Engine" in Swahili—by his training partners. Mutai was beginning to see why. Each time he attacked, Mosop responded. Mutai was determined to shake him, to run alone, to feel the Spirit course through him. Again and again, Mutai pressed. Again and again, Mosop roared back. With both men trying to kill one another, the split times approached the supernatural. "There was not one kilometer when we relaxed the pace," Mutai remembers, fireworks behind his eyes as he recalls the battle. "We were fighting!"

In the final few hundred meters, Mutai made one more move as the pair rounded the bend onto Boylston Street and ended his rival's challenge for good. The gap grew. Two meters, five meters, ten meters. He hit the line, arms raised to each side, as the announcer on the course screamed, astonishment in his voice, "In two-oh-three *FLAT* . . ."

In fact, Mutai finished in 2:03:02. Those numbers would color the rest of his career. The time was worth life-changing money. He received $225,000 there and then—$150,000 for the win, $50,000 for the world's best time, and $25,000 for a new course record. There was also the question of what those numbers would allow Mutai to command in future appearance fees. He was now the fastest marathoner in history. There was talk of a quarter of a million dollars for him just to show up to his next race. He was also well on the way to a possible World Marathon Majors jackpot of half a million. And then Adidas, his shoe sponsor, would want to reward him.

In human terms, however, the time threatened to break him. The double asterisk hung over the performance. Not only was Boston ineligible for a world record, but people carried on and on about the wind. Those conversations infuriated him, although you never would have known from his equitable demeanor.

"I tried to enjoy it," he remembers. "But . . ." The right words don't come. "It was painful. It's like, you are climbing a tree, and you nearly reach the top, and then you drop down. And now I have to climb it again."

———

Mutai's injury was internal, and he nursed it privately. He had, after all, won a Major for the first time. He had also located the key to unlocking races: more aggression, earlier. These were successes worth celebrating. He also knew that the only cure for his ailment would be more victories on the roads. There was nothing to do but go back to work.

Meanwhile, he could not help noticing that his life at home was changing beyond recognition. He was a father now to a lively, beautiful little girl named Michelle, whom he adored. He put gold studs in his daughter's ears and moved his family into a large, two-story house in Elgon View, the most prestigious area of Eldoret. He bought rental properties in town and invested in farmland. He drove expensive off-road vehicles, whose flatbeds were often filled to bursting with training pals or with bundles of vegetables from his farm. He wore better clothes.

However, Mutai knew how many runners' heads had been turned by money, and he still continued to live in humble circumstances in Kapng'tuny six days a week. By 2011, he had moved into a tiny cottage halfway down a muddy hill with three other athletes. His house was flanked by fields containing Friesian cows on one side, chickens on the other, and three fly-ridden "long-drop" outhouses a few yards from the front door. There was no running water. When Mutai or his housemates wanted to wash, eat, clean, or do laundry, they walked outside to the well, lowered a bucket, and drew the water with a rope.

Mutai shared cooking duties with his friends. They prepared meals while crouching over a camping stove in the cool larder-cum-kitchen at the back of the house. Often the dish would be simple: *ugali* with *managu*, a nettly vegetable that they fried in a skillet. Sometimes they would cook pasta. Very occasionally, they would eat meat.

Mutai was a rich man—a dollar millionaire at least. He didn't need to live like this. Considered in purely economic terms, his life in Kapng'tuny was a façade, a playact. At his large, well-appointed house in Eldoret, Mutai would undertake few of the domestic chores that he did in camp. It would be women's work, conducted out of sight by his wife and female relations.

But out here in the sticks there were different rules. The men looked after themselves. Self-sufficiency was not an inconvenience, he believed, but a training aid. The idea was to live humbly and work hard, with few distractions, in a community dedicated to punishing rituals. Mutai had the money to lord it over his colleagues, but he chose not to do so, for pragmatic as well as ethical reasons. He said he needed them as much as they needed him.

Mutai's tiny room in the cottage—perhaps eight or ten square feet—contained a single bed. There was a CD player and radio on the bedside table, and a makeshift clothesline strung from one corner of the room to the other. Flies buzzed around a bulb that hung unshaded from the ceiling. One wall was decorated with newspaper clippings of his recent triumphs. On the adjacent wall was a token of affection from his wife—a poster, on which the following English text was written in loopy calligraphy: "My Darling, I promise to always be there for you in favourable and unfavourable situations, anywhere, anytime. Know that you hold a special place in my heart."

Sometimes Mutai's wife and two daughters, who lived in some luxury in Eldoret, came to visit. Mutai recalled with a chuckle that his oldest daughter asked him why he would live in such a place, in such a manner. "I tell her that we like it here, we enjoy it," said Mutai. "But she don't believe it."

As Wanjiru's story proved, the pressures on men of wealth and property in Kenya are significant. Here, in a dead-end town, miles from anywhere, Mutai went about his business largely untroubled. The only bother he endured was from the many drunkards in the town who tugged on his arm for money when he shopped for groceries, or as he walked to the teahouse for *chapattis*. But they were easily ignored. When Mutai was in the cottage he swept and scrubbed, or relaxed in front of cheap Chinese DVDs dubbed into Swahili. At night, he would sometimes drive off to the nearby village of Torongo with a few friends for a *nyama choma* barbecue—a Kenyan delicacy. Most of all, he ran.

———

Mutai's program was a simple one. An early run, before dawn, was followed by a breakfast of chai—the weak, milky, sugary tea favored by Kenyans—and bread. While he lived in the cottage on the hill, the milk for the tea was brought to his house in a plastic jug by a schoolboy named Renson Kiprotich. Cheeky as a squirrel, with a gap-toothed smile and knock-knees, he was the smartest boy in the village, and already a grade ahead at school. He spoke immaculate old-fashioned English.

One morning when I was staying in the cottage with Mutai and his fellow athletes, Renson knocked on the door.

"Let me greet these gentlemen," he said to Mutai. Then, extending his hand to me, he said: "Hello, white man."

Mutai giggled. The boy was twelve years old. Renson's English was better than his own.

Renson performed the milk run every day before school. His reward was a little money and breakfast with Mutai and his housemates—a privilege of which his schoolmates were justly envious. Despite his precocious academic ability, Renson was not planning to go to high school, because his parents could not afford the school fees. Mutai took obvious pleasure in being able to do something for the kid. Breakfast time was a sweet scene: three runners with a total of eight big-money marathon wins between them, huddled up in a cold, smoky room with the school nerd.

At around 9 a.m., the athletes began their most serious workout of the day. In other parts of running country, "speedwork"—the interspersing of periods of fast and slow running—was often done on the track. But Kapng'tuny was nowhere near a track, and anyway, Mutai saw no need to run in circles. Hills, he believed, "stayed in the legs" longer than running on flat ground. Every session—speedwork, *Fartlek*, long runs, easy runs—took place on God's own racetrack: the dirt roads of Skyland.

Many sessions were savage. At one I witnessed, five dozen athletes convened at the edge of Kapng'tuny for speedwork. The workout started with a twenty-minute warm-up run, up and over hills, gradually increasing in pace. About ten minutes into the warm-up, the group passed a farm laborer on his way to work. The man was about fifty years old, with a lean figure, a beard, and a soul patch. He was wearing a tattered auburn suit with black office shoes missing their laces. Glad of the company, he ran more than a mile with Mutai's group before dropping out. Nobody mentioned his presence, either during the training session or afterward. It seemed utterly unremarkable that a middle-aged workingman could keep pace with some of the world's greatest athletes.

After twenty minutes' jogging, the session could begin in earnest. The plan was to run eighteen sprints of two minutes each with a minute of slow jogging in between. Including the warm-up, the athletes would cover more than 13 miles in total: up and down hills, at altitude.

As a senior athlete, Mutai took his leadership role seriously. (He had, for instance, learned sign language to communicate with the two deaf runners in his group.) As the workout gained momentum, he took his place at the head of the pack. Wearing a red top and black shorts, he ensured that the sprints were fast enough for his liking. It was thrilling to watch. Sometimes Mutai and the strongest men would sprint so fast that they overtook the 50cc motorcycle I was riding. As the session wore on, large gaps appeared in the group. Some athletes stopped altogether after five or six sprints. Some hung on, farther back. A group of around eight athletes managed to complete the session at the fastest pace—many of them already winners at marathons like Tokyo and Paris.

At the end of the workout, the boss remarked, "Now you see why I need these men."

———

But what Mutai needed—really needed—was always something of a puzzle. Certainly it was more than success. Or perhaps he configured success in a different way than his fellow athletes, for whom marathon wins and the accompanying riches were, to use the Lutheran argot, visible signs of election.

Mutai desired more than medals or money, although both were important to him. He wanted to be validated, redeemed in some way. This diagnostic lack was revealed in every punishment he meted out to himself on the dirt roads. He was not satisfied, could not be satisfied. It was a curse, of sorts—to be so great, and accept it so little—but also, one suspected, the font of his greatness.

When he spoke about what drove him, it would often be at the end of a day in which he had trained well and his body seemed purged. Collapsed on a sofa, half-watching the television news, he would offer a clue. One night in Kapng'tuny, Mutai said that during his ascendant period, as victory followed victory, he had waited to hear something—an acceptance? an apology?—from his father, who had blighted his childhood and chastised his choice of profession. But none came. Mutai said there had been "only silence" on the difficult subject of the past. Rather, his whole family—including his father—chose to celebrate his successes with him. Geoffrey accepted their attentions. In fact, he rejoiced in them. A long time before he made any money from running, Mutai had asked his father how much it would cost to fix the roof of the old man's house in Rongai. Now, with the money secured, he commissioned the necessary work.

This might seem like a profound act of forgiveness. To Mutai, however, there was no other path. He understood where he had come from, and that to break familial bonds would be a derogation of his identity. "I don't want revenge," he said. "My parents are my parents. I can't change it. I don't have any other father."

To illustrate his point, Mutai explained a curious aspect of Kalenjin names. His father is called Andrew Kimutai Koech. Geoffrey's full name is Geoffrey Kiprono Mutai. Men do not pass surnames on to each other down a long line, as happens in Western countries. Instead, the surname of the son is drawn from the middle name of the father, minus the prefix: a one-generation transaction. So these two men, Geoffrey explained, were coupled not only by biology, but by nomenclature. They shared that filial link—Kimutai to Mutai—and nothing would ever alter that relationship.

The same night, Mutai told another story about his father. Once, after he had won a race in Europe, Mutai heard that his family had held a party in Rongai in his honor. At this gathering, his father had become emotional, almost tearful, before telling the other guests that "this boy, he has always been working hard." Mutai was told this anecdote secondhand, by a sibling. His father had never summoned the courage to say those words to his first-born face-to-face.

"One day," said Mutai, "we will talk."

———

After Boston, Mutai wanted to race in New York in November. The obvious choice for an athlete wishing to fortify his credentials as the fastest in history would be Berlin, where most world records are set. But having been disappointed in Germany the previous year, he did not want to run there again so soon. In particular, he had no desire to escort Makau—who would surely be invited to Berlin, as reigning champion—once more to the finish line. What's more, he had never run New York before. It was a tough course, with a tradition of hard-fought races and no pacemakers. If he won there, nobody could be in any doubt about his achievement.

On November 6, 2011, a bitter, sunny day in New York, the field was stacked with talent. Among the favorites were Emmanuel Mutai, who had won the 2011 London Marathon in April in a course record of 2:04:40, and Tsegaye Kebede, the tiny Ethiopian who had beaten Emmanuel in the 2010 London Marathon and lost the battle with Sammy Wanjiru in Chicago later the same year.

Geoffrey killed them all in what may be the greatest performance in the history of the marathon. At 20 miles, there were still seven athletes in the lead group, including all the favorites and Meb Keflezighi, the last American to win the New York Marathon, in 2009. It was at this moment that Mutai decided to break the pack with a sledgehammer. He ran the three-mile section between mile 20 and mile 23 in 13 minutes and 35 seconds—an average of 4:31 per mile. (That's preposterously fast—if you ran a whole marathon at 4:31 per mile, you'd finish in 1 hour, 58 minutes.) Although Mutai's pace dropped a little after his assault, he maintained his aggression all the way to the end of the race. Nobody but he survived. Mutai crossed the line more than a minute ahead of his nearest rival and more than two and a half minutes ahead of the course record, in 2:05:06—a previously unthinkable time in New York. He raised his arms high and pumped his biceps, and for perhaps the only time anyone could remember, he looked halfway satisfied.

In the commentary booth, Toni Reavis talked about what Mutai's run meant. Only four men before him had ever won Boston and New York in the same year. None of those champions had ever broken course records in both marathons. Mutai's run, said the commentator, had silenced the chatter around Boston. Using his feet to talk, the Kenyan had told the world: "Kids, that was *real*. And here's proof."

For others in the road-running world, Mutai's run changed

everything. He had taken a combined total of more than five minutes out of the course records at two unpaced marathons, and had done so in a way that left people dumbstruck—with sustained bouts of aggression from a long way out. It was as if he had discovered a new sport.

Renato Canova, a white-haired Italian coach who wears wraparound sunglasses whatever the weather and has worked with many of the top Kenyan marathoners, was overwhelmed by the brilliance of Mutai's run in New York. He believed that had Mutai run Berlin in the kind of form he showed in New York, he might have set a time of 2:02:20 or 2:02:30, which would have been more than a minute faster than Makau's world record. Canova also argued that the wind was not as much of a factor in Boston as others had made out. The breeze, he said, came from the side as much as the back. He believed Mutai and Mosop had not been given the credit they deserved for their incredible times.

A few months after Mutai's New York triumph, another Italian coach was still scratching his head. After Wanjiru's death, Claudio Berardelli continued to work with some excellent elite runners, including the future New York and London women's champion, Priscah Jeptoo, and the men's prospect Stanley Biwott. He had been in Kenya seven years when Geoffrey Mutai completed his astonishing 2011, and he admitted that those performances had left him "a little bit confused."

One cool morning in February 2012, while driving his Toyota Hilux along the Nangili road, just outside of Eldoret, and watching his elite athletes on an early morning run, he said: "It was like, all of a sudden, the marathon has become shorter. Like the ten-thousand-meter philosophy and the half-marathon philosophy have been combined. . . . The marathon is now, 'Well, it's a couple of hours running, and we can push as hard as we can.' Before, everyone was scared. They waited until thirty kilometers. You didn't do anything [before then], you just stayed quiet, relaxed, because you might finish your fuel."

———

Berardelli was not the only one whose ideas were upended by Mutai. The new approach to marathon running was even changing the way the shoe companies were designing their sneakers. At Adidas headquarters in Germany, the designers Andy Barr and George Vontsolos had long thought about the ways in which footwear affects marathon times. It was in their interests for the world record to be broken by a man wearing their shoes, and they were quick to point out that in 2007, 2008, and 2011, an Adidas athlete had done so.

Before Mutai and the golden year of marathoning in 2011, the key to their thinking had been to make the shoes lightweight. Research conducted on behalf of Adidas in the lead-up to the 2012 Olympic Games concluded that saving 100 grams of weight on the foot translated into a 1 percent energy saving for an athlete. This finding related to one of the most interesting aspects of the genetic debate about the Kenyan running phenomenon.

As a group, Kalenjin runners are extremely slender below the knee. This physiological trait is believed to be connected to their heritage in the baking-hot Nile Valley. Thinner limbs cool quicker. Even though the Kalenjin now live at altitude, they have retained their slender legs. One study showed that Kalenjin elite runners had 5 percent longer legs and 12 percent lighter legs than a group of Swedish elite runners. In his outstanding book, *The Sports Gene,* David Epstein explains: "Weight that is far out on the limbs is called 'distal weight,' and the less of it a distance runner has, the better."

A light shoe, therefore, is paramount to marathoners who are already as sleek as racing greyhounds. In the past decade, most companies produced racing flats that felt like ballet shoes. But recently, the Adidas team decided to reconsider its design priorities. From talking to Geoffrey Mutai, Haile Gebrselassie, and Wilson Kipsang, the top marathon runners in the Adidas stable, the designers had a surprising revelation. The way they were thinking about racing shoes ran counter to what their athletes wanted.

"Originally, our position was that they wanted something that's basically like running barefoot," said Barr. "Less than a hundred grams, not a lot of cushioning. And what the athletes wanted was almost the exact opposite. What the guys said to us was that the way the marathon's being run now, they need to get to twenty miles with as minimal fatigue as possible. They described to us what they needed: almost like a trainer [a sneaker] up until twenty miles, and then when the hammer goes down at twenty, twenty-one, twenty-two miles, they want something that's a pure racing flat."

In the past few years, Adidas has attempted to solve this problem by moving away from the "barefoot" idea to a more cushioned racing shoe. It's still light, but it's bulkier than other racing flats used by athletes and has what is known in sneaker design terms as a higher "heel-to-toe drop."

"The market almost went in a completely different direction, in that they were going lower to the ground, lower heel-to-toe drop," said Barr. "Look at a Nike flat, look at a Brooks flat. If you look at most flats out there, they'll be lower to the ground. We have a formula that goes against the conventional wisdom."

In recent years, this kind of thinking amounts to heresy. Since the publication of Christopher McDougall's *Born to Run,* and the explosion of the barefoot running movement, the training shoe industry has moved toward less cushioning to encourage a more minimalist approach. The debate about the benefits of cushioning in training shoes is somewhat toxic in running circles. Suffice it to say that for every barefoot evangelist there are many scientists who are unconvinced that running barefoot, or with minimal protection, helps prevent injury. A 2013 scientific paper noted that studies into this area were "in their infancy" and that "the link between barefoot running and injury or performance remains tenuous and speculative."

In any case, what the designers at Adidas discovered, and what any visitor to Ethiopian or Kenyan running country will notice, is that professional runners like protection. Yes, many of the kids who grow up to be marathon superstars spend a significant time running in bare feet, and this unshod childhood almost certainly contributes to their preeminence as distance runners. But as soon as East Africans can afford training shoes, they buy them. It is inconceivable that they could cover the miles they do as professional athletes without a little cushioning.

Marathon runners also believe that shoes make a difference to marathon times. Haile, in particular, is a sneakerhead. He believes that shoe technology is a much more significant driver of the marathon world record progression than any developments in training. Granted, he is paid a significant sum of money by Adidas, and his views may be colored by that relationship. But he has also broken the world record twice.

"All sport is helped by technology," he said. "If someone says to me it's not technology, it's the ability of the athletes, no, no. . . . I've been running the last twenty-two years. I know the shoes in the late eighties, early nineties. Every year, the shoes that we have completely change. And now I'm thinking what will be in the future."

So are the shoe companies. Adidas now uses a proprietary substance called Boost foam in their shoes that they believe returns more energy to the athlete than the traditional EVA substance used in sneakers. A University of Calgary study agreed with Adidas on this point: Boost foam outscored EVA by 1 percent in their trials. Marathon results, too, seem to be going in Adidas's favor, with the three fastest times of 2013 run by their athletes—which may or may not be a coincidence.

Barr had assumed that the new technology would simply be a racing aid for the elite athletes. But when he showed the new Boost shoes to Geoffrey Mutai, the athlete's first question was not whether the technology would allow him to race faster, but whether it would allow him to train harder. The next step for the Adidas designers might be to take a further step back from convention and design a bulky, super-cushioned training shoe for their best runners.

———

Far away from the laboratory, out on the dirt roads, Coach Berardelli was still at a loss as to what had changed so suddenly in the marathon. Bodies could not evolve so quickly. The coach eventually landed upon a simple answer. It was, he said, "mentality." Haile started the development in 2008, by running a 62-minute first half in Berlin on the way to his world record.

Before that run, it was a "crazy" idea to go out in 62 minutes dead—a surefire way to lose a race. But after the Kenyans saw Haile in Berlin, they realized they could run big personal bests by being more aggressive earlier in the race. By the end of the decade and the beginning of the next, that attitude had percolated into training. Instead of pounding out endless slow miles, the best runners worked on a new theory: high volume, high intensity. It was agony, and it worked.

By 2011, the best marathoners were all prepared for a fast opening—somewhere between 61:45 and 62 minutes. It didn't scare them. But what Geoffrey Mutai did that was so different from almost everyone else was to use a rapid, even first half as merely a prologue to an explosion of speed later in the race. The change wasn't made with exact pacing calculations in mind, Berardelli thought, but rather by "feeling the body" in the second half of the race and just deciding to attack. It was the absence of fear—the opposite of fear.

The problem for Berardelli was that understanding the change was not the same as being able to respond to it. He needed to look deeper. In Kenya, the prevailing wisdom about the marathon had been that a runner's energy sources were divided, more or less, into "sugars" and "fats." Sugars were better to run on than fats but would only take you so far in a race—perhaps 35km—before they were used up. So it was thought to be impossible to run the whole race at full steam—on "sugars." This was the origin of the Kenyan adage: "The race begins at thirty-five." And it is one of the many reasons why athletes used to hang on, running steady, so as not to burn themselves out too much before the final stretch.

What Mutai seemed to be doing was preserving his energy for

a long time in a race and then scorching a trail in the latter half. He seemed to able to run on fats before he ran on sugars.

"Of course," said Berardelli, with his voice somewhere between rueful and awed, "you can train people to run faster. But not everyone can run the new way. They are not capable, genetically. Not everyone in Kenya can run like Geoffrey Mutai."

That statement prompted a twofold question. First, why couldn't Americans, or Brits, or Japanese set their minds to running in this new way? What, in other words, made Kenyans so special? And, second, why was Mutai, at that moment, better than all of them?

Chapter Seven

Not Everyone Can Run Like Geoffrey Mutai

V INCENZO LANCINI, a physiotherapist from Brescia, Italy, believes he knows the answer to the first question: feet. He's
obsessed with the feet of Kenyan runners, and has taken hundreds of photographs of them as mementos. He reveres these
appendages as a music lover might revere Lang Lang's sinuous
fingers. For him, feet hold the key to understanding the dominance of Kenya—and, more generally, East Africa—over the
marathon world.

Lancini first came to running country in the early 2000s to
work with the Rosa group's top athletes, including the three-time
London Marathon winner, Martin Lel. It was when he was mas-
saging Lel that he first noticed his feet were freakish. Hypertro-
phied muscles bulged out of them, as on a bodybuilder's torso.
Their arches were elastic and strong. Lancini had worked on all
kinds of athletes from all kinds of sports, including European

runners, and he possessed a sensual literacy when it came to understanding their bodies. But he had never felt or seen anything like these feet. They were, in his words, like "trampolines"—when they hit the ground, they returned energy to the runner in extraordinary ways.

Lancini asked if he could take a photograph of Lel's feet. The bemused runner acceded to the request. While Lancini was wondering about the specific ways in which such powerful feet might be important to a runner, he started noticing that the Kenyan runners he was treating also had unusually strong muscles on either side of their spines: long, strong, cylindrical, and rounded "like the pipes of an organ."

Connections started to form. Lancini reasoned that these highly responsive, superstrength feet were steadying the runners as they motored along. They were acting, in his words, both as "trampolines" and as "grounding tools." He explained that every time a Kenyan runner strikes with his foot, it's as if he is driving an antenna into the road that will then fling him forward. As Lancini's hardworking fingers understood, all of the best Kenyans possessed a strong and flexible chain from those muscular feet through the abdominal corset to the trophic chain of muscles in the back and neck. But, in the Italian physiotherapist's mind, it all began with the feet. Simply put, a Kenyan's feet propelled him faster than other athletes', with a smaller loss of energy.

Lancini believes this special quality is developed by the large amount of time that Kenyan runners spend barefoot as children and as young teenagers. (However, if you watch a top adult runner like Geoffrey Mutai train, on uneven, rough roads, you realize how micro-training these foot and lower leg muscles continues when Kenyan runners put on shoes. Mutai doesn't spend a minute of his working day on a flat surface, and so his muscles are always working to balance and respond.)

"They learn to listen with their feet," says Lancini.

——

As Lancini acknowledges, feet can only be part of the answer. There are so many factors involved in athletic success, and many of the most significant are not physiological. Science can't give us all the answers to Geoffrey Mutai because it can't allow us access to the secrets of his heart or the specifics of his upbringing. But it can give us clues. There are things science can *test*, aspects it can measure. Moreover, in the Kenyan runners, sports science has been gifted the most extraordinary sample of geographically concentrated athletic dominance in any sport.

What's so intriguing about Kenya's success at long distances, and what makes the scientists who study the reasons behind that success so excited, is that their champions almost uniformly hail from one tribe: the Kalenjin. Although there are exceptions, like Sammy Wanjiru—a Kikuyu—it's a good bet that if you see a Kenyan winning a marathon, he or she will come from a fairly small patch of the globe, in the highlands at the western edge of the Rift Valley.

You can narrow down the profile, and the biography, still further. Almost all successful runners were brought up on arable smallholdings in large families in modest circumstances. They walked and ran to school, barefoot. As teenagers, they helped out on farms. When the men entered adolescence, they endured brutal circumcision ceremonies—after which, as part of the same ritual, they were forced to fend for themselves for days and weeks at a time outside the relative comfort of their family home.

Kenya is a poor country. But up in running country the soil is rich, and an average Kalenjin smallholding family can grow enough to eat. In fact, the diet of the Kalenjin is nearly perfect for an endurance athlete: it consists mostly of *ugali,* a starchy carbohydrate, with vegetables and, occasionally, meat. All this is washed down with buckets of sweet, milky tea.

An average young rural Kalenjin is active, and eats nutritiously but sparingly. There isn't much disposable income, so shoes are a luxury. His feet become used to the feel of the earth, and the tendons in his ankle strengthen. He also lives his scampering life at altitude. Most areas of Kenyan running country sit above 7,000 feet. Such an existence leads a future athlete to have a greater oxygen-carrying capacity at sea level. As an adult, his heart and lungs are a more efficient engine. The question is not one of lung *capacity,* as such, but of the power of those lungs to ingest oxygen. A number of studies have shown that the lungs of athletes who are exposed to altitude over long periods of time have a greater "diffusing capacity" than those of sea-level dwellers. The surface area of the lung where the gas exchange occurs can be as much as 50 percent greater in altitude dwellers.

As David Epstein explains in *The Sports Gene,* there are many nuances to the effect of altitude on the development of athletes. For one thing, it is preferable to be born at altitude rather than simply to train there. Those who are born high develop larger lungs than those who are born at sea level. This trait has little to do with genes because it applies equally to people with sea-level ancestry who happen to be born and spend their childhood at altitude as it does to the children of Himalayan farmers.

Some populations respond much better to living and training at altitude than others. Their responsiveness appears to be connected to how long the population has lived high. For instance, Epstein cites the work of Cynthia Beall, a physical anthropology professor at Case Western Reserve University in Cleveland, who tested two Ethiopian groups, the Amhara and the Oromo, both of whom lived at altitude, for their levels of hemoglobin, the oxygen-transport protein in red blood cells. The Amhara possessed low hemoglobin levels even at high altitudes. The Oromo, on the other hand, had high hemoglobin levels even at much lower altitudes. What accounts for this difference is hard to discern at first glance. Both groups live at a roughly similar altitude. But whereas the Amhara have resided in their current location for millennia, the Oromo moved up to the highlands only centuries ago. The Oromo are, effectively, lowlanders who live high.

"A helpful combination," writes Epstein, "is to have sea-level ancestry—so that hemoglobin can elevate quickly upon training at altitude—but to be born at altitude, in order to develop larger lung surface area, and then to live and train in the sweet spot [between six and nine thousand feet above sea level]. This is exactly the story of legions of Kalenjin Kenyans and Oromo Ethiopians."

In fact, the story is slightly more complicated with the Kalenjin. All of them moved from the Nile Valley to the Rift Valley centuries ago, but some, such as the Nandi and the Kipsigis, have spent longer at altitude than the other Kalenjin subtribes, such as the Pokot and the Keiyo, who moved high in large numbers within the past half century. The crucial point is that they are all, physiologically, valley people who live up the mountain.

——

These accidents of history and culture dominate much of the conversation about Kenyan running. The argument goes that an active, altitudinous life allows any inherent athletic talent in a Kalenjin boy or girl to emerge. But this is also a story about numbers. Thousands of Kalenjin men and women are currently in training. All of them know the path to success and the rewards available to the very best runners, because Kalenjin athletes have competed against, and beaten, the rest of the world for fifty years.

At the Tokyo Olympics in 1964, Wilson Kiprugut became the first Kenyan to win an Olympic medal for the newly independent country when he took bronze in the 800m. Four years later, the Kenyans—including their new superstar of track and field, Kip Keino—won three golds, four silvers, and a bronze in middle- and long-distance running events in the thin air of Mexico City. Indeed, African men won every event over 800m at the 1968 Games.

Athletics in this period was still defiantly amateur. Success at the Olympics was a boon for a newly minted country but was unlikely to profoundly change the lives of the runners involved. In the next decade, however, Kenyans began to see running as a means to escape rural poverty. U.S. colleges began to cherry-pick Kenyan athletes for track scholarships. Meet directors started to invite the new African stars to events in Europe. Over the period in which Kenya boycotted the Olympics (1976 and 1980), these relationships sustained a number of top athletes who might have had no other outlet for their talent.

Meanwhile, back in the thin air of Iten, a village perched on the edge of the Rift Valley in the heart of Kalenjin country, the foundations were being laid for a fortress of distance running. In 1976, a young Irishman named Brother Colm O'Connell arrived to begin a teaching career at St. Patrick's, a school with a reputation for sports that was founded by the Patrician Brothers, an Irish order devoted to education, in the final years before Kenyan independence.

O'Connell was replacing a twenty-one-year-old Brit named Peter Foster, whose brother Brendan would win bronze in the 10,000m at the Montreal Olympics later that summer. Peter coached the St. Patrick's track team using training techniques he had picked up from his and Brendan's mentor in Newcastle, England, a man named Stan Long.

"Stan basically taught us *Fartlek* [interval training], hillwork, long runs on a Sunday, that sort of thing," Foster told me. "That's all I did with the Kenyans. It was a bit of a revolution, because before that they would just try and run as hard as they possibly could for the same distance every time they went out."

When O'Connell arrived, he was told he was Foster's replacement. O'Connell had never watched a track meet, let alone coached one. (His expertise was mostly in Gaelic football, an unpopular sport in the Rift Valley.) But he caught on quickly. Using Foster's ideas and his own intuition, he began to coach the children how to run faster. It was not a complicated process. Like a prospector who plants a pick in the desert and finds himself drenched in oil, he realized pretty soon that he had struck athletic paydirt. Many of his pupils were not only in possession of considerable athletic talent; they were also prepared to work. All

O'Connell had to do was to give them direction. As he often says of his success, "The secret is: there is no secret."

St. Patrick's became an athletic powerhouse, winning countless school titles. Soon it began to attract talented kids from all over running country. Such was its reputation that in 1986, O'Connell was asked by the national track federation to select the Kenyan team for the World Junior Championships. Not knowing any better, he picked nine St. Patrick's students. All of them came back with medals.

The Patrician Brother is now an avuncular, potbellied man in his mid-sixties, and he has retired from the school where he made his name. He still coaches professional athletes, like the 800m Olympic champion and world record holder David Rudisha, and continues to hold summer camps for talented children. Nearly forty years after he arrived in Kenya, he can justifiably claim to be one of the most successful track coaches of all time. Twenty-five world champions and five Olympic gold medalists have come through his programs.

O'Connell has witnessed, and to some extent driven, the Kenyan distance running phenomenon. When he arrived in Iten, he remembers it being a "dot on the map," a remote village with little importance in Kenyan or international life. Now people all over the world recognize it as an athletic mecca. Mo Farah and Paula Radcliffe have trained there, hoping that the magic of the red-dirt roads will rub off. At certain times of day, one can't move for groups of runners pounding off down a dirt track. Most of these men and women don't make a cent from running. But some in their midst do make money, plenty of it. For poor people with few other lucrative prospects, there is a powerful motivation to run fast.

——

Kenya began producing outstanding running results in the 1970s and 1980s, mostly on the track. Until recently, however, the marathon was an unattractive distance for many Kenyan runners. It was something track athletes did at the end of their careers, when they were past their prime but still had "miles in the legs." But from the 1980s onward Kenyans began to understand they could change their lives with one big run. Joseph Nzau was the first Kenyan to win a major marathon in America, the 1983 Chicago Marathon, but he was based in the United States, at the University of Wyoming. The first real Kenyan stars of the international marathon circuit were Ibrahim Hussein, who won three Honolulu Marathons, three Boston Marathons, and one New York City Marathon, and Douglas Wakiihuri, an Olympic silver medalist who then won both London and New York.

By the 1990s, managers and agents from Europe and America began to arrive in Kenya, scouring Kalenjin country for talent. Little by little, an economy developed. Promising athletes would sign with an agent or management team, who would organize for them to compete in races abroad, taking a 15 percent cut of any money earned. At this time, Kenyans still competed more often on the track than the road. The prize money available was not enough to tempt East Africans to wreck their bodies, twice a year, when they could win decent money for any number of five- and ten-thousand-meter races. There was also, several Kenyans say, a widespread belief that running too many marathons could make a man infertile.

By the 2000s, the money in track began to be eclipsed by the money available in the marathon, and whatever reservations

Kenyans felt about running 26.2 miles were allayed. Now, in Kalenjin country, there's only one game in town, and everyone wants a piece. If you believe you have any talent as a runner, you train your guts out to see if you can make it. (And most of them seem to believe they have talent. Coach Berardelli says it's a peculiarity of Kalenjins that they possess utter faith that "anybody can run—it's only a question of training.") In the village of Iten, in the forests of Kaptagat, and in the backroads of Kapsabet, the dirt roads teem with young men and women, running in groups. They train twice or three times a day. There are few joggers; casual running barely exists. In Kenya, there is no time for dilettantes. You either want to be a professional or you work in some other way.

If you're really enterprising, you do both. A story: One day, I went to a tumbledown teahouse in Iten with a friend of mine, Elias Maindi, a two-oh-eight guy. Elias needed milk for his chai, and so we walked across the road to the teahouse. As we were buying the milk we heard a strange scraping noise out back. We went outside to find a young man working a small knife into a severed and charred cow's head. I asked him what he was doing. He explained that although all the best cuts from the cow had been sold, he was salvaging the meat and bones from the head to make a soup for his family, and that it was going to be delicious. Eventually he went back to his work and Elias and I went home for tea.

The next day, I was at the nearby track at Kamariny, watching Wilson Kipsang's group complete a speedwork session. This ramshackle facility is the center of Iten's running scene. It has cracked wooden bleachers on one side and a row of low cottages that are often rented by athletes on the other. In the middle of the oval is a dusty soccer field that is sometimes the scene of raucously supported inter-school matches that seem to feature many more than eleven players per side.

Groups of athletes work out on the dirt running surface here every morning. On that particular day, it was a scrum. There may have been sixty runners using the track at the same time. Meanwhile, several dozen athletes who had either just finished or were just about to begin their training milled and stretched on the soccer field. I was just about to leave Kamariny when a young man I didn't recognize approached. He told me how his training had gone that morning—how many repetitions of 400 meters he had done, and how his hamstring felt. I listened to him with evidently a somewhat blank expression on my face. It seemed clear that he knew who I was, but I couldn't place him. Eventually he put me out of my misery.

"You don't know me?" he asked.

No, I had to admit.

"But you saw me yesterday!" he said, laughing.

And then I remembered. It was the cow's head soup guy. Somehow I hadn't pegged him as an athlete, and he'd never mentioned it. But then I remembered that in Iten, everyone is a runner.

It's not only a question of large numbers of people, some of whom have extraordinary talent, training hard. In order to succeed at international competitions, Kenyans need to be on the startline. Since the 1990s, when the Kenyan authorities relaxed the rules about foreign agents coming into the country to scout for talent, there has been a pipeline, spiriting the best runners to the best events in Europe and America.

At its best, this system makes people richer and happier,

At its worst, the system is abusive. There are agents with bad reputations. Some junior athletes tell stories of being taken to Europe and encouraged to run as many as five 10km or half-marathon races in a month and being injured for months afterward.

That is the worst of the system. Most agents, however, are well-intentioned. If you are a young Kenyan runner, your first priority is to find an agent or manager who can help you race *outside* and bring home dollars or euros. The agent's job is to facilitate that process while constantly keeping an eye out for the next Geoffrey Mutai. This system is imprecise, but there's scant chance of genuine talent slipping away.

When Geoffrey Kamworor—now the world half-marathon champion, and Haile's pick for a future marathon world record holder—won the Mara half marathon in Kenya, having just graduated from high school, he was spotted by a coach named Richard Meto, who works alongside Patrick Sang, a former Olympic silver medalist and now the coach of several top marathoners, including Emmanuel Mutai. On Meto's suggestion, Sang took a look at Kipsang, and recommended to Jos Hermens and Global Sports that they sign the kid. That's how it works: run well in a local race and someone will be watching.

The question remains of where the talent comes from in the first place. It's not enough simply to point at the numbers of people who take up the sport in the Rift Valley. If, for some reason, the people of Lithuania were suddenly seized by the marathon bug and decided to train in vast numbers from a young age, then Lithuania might eventually produce a few more elite marathon runners. But it's highly doubtful it would become a powerhouse of distance running, like Kenya.

The complete domination of marathoning by East Africans prompts a difficult question. When it comes to the long distances, are East Africans genetically superior?

——

The science of genes is swelling, rapidly changing, and forbiddingly complicated. But there are only certain aspects of the science that are immediately pertinent to the understanding of the East African distance running phenomenon. Largely, it is a debate about nature versus nurture.

It is now more than a decade since the Human Genome Project completed its work in 2003, finding around 20,500 individual genes. The mapping of the HGP allowed us to see the building blocks of our DNA—the most basic elements of how we are made, and the means by which information is passed from one generation to another.

At first it was believed that *individual* genes might hold the clues not only to disease but to other human traits such as speed or obesity. In some cases, that has proved to be true. One can identify the genes responsible for diseases like cystic fibrosis or sickle-cell anemia. There are also identifiable athletic genes, or "gene variants," that have been the focus of much study by sports scientists over the past few years. Almost all Olympic sprinters, for instance, carry the "correct" version of the ACTN3 gene, which influences fast-twitch muscle fibers.

Yannis Pitsiladis is one scientist for whom this area of study has proved irresistible. He is fascinated in particular by the connection between our genetic makeup and our athletic ability. A garrulous man in his late forties whose childhood was spent in Australia and South Africa, and who now holds a post at the

University of Brighton on the south coast of England, he has devoted a large portion of his adult life to answering the question of why East Africans are so good at distance running.

When we met in Eldoret, in 2012, he was midway through a months-long project in the Rift Valley, testing Kalenjin schoolchildren for their activity levels and lung capacity. He was also conducting tests on elite runners for any kind of "performance gene." In one experiment, Pitsiladis tested Kalenjin runners for the ACE and the ACTN3 genes, which are both known to be associated with athletic excellence. He wanted to discover whether there was a single gene, or gene variant, that differentiated Kenyan runners from the rest of the world's elite. But so far, there had been no eureka moment.

At our meeting, Pitsiladis was definitive. He said that he believed there was no genetic basis for Kenya's dominance of distance running. Based on what he understood about their genetic makeup, there was little to distinguish Kenyans, or the Kalenjin, as a population, from the rest of the world's populations. Rather, he said, we should look to all those lifestyle and socioeconomic elements—the bare feet, the altitude, the diet, the *desire*—for an answer to their dominance of the sport.

But in a recent coauthored paper, Pitsiladis allowed the caveat that it was possible future studies might reverse his position. He still believed that Kenyan running success was not a "genetically mediated phenomenon." But *if* Kenyan success was later found to be explicable by genetics, the answer would most likely reside in the interplay of various genes, rather than in one particular "performance gene."

Ross Tucker of the Sports Science Institute of South Africa takes issue with some of Pitsiladis's methods and conclusions.

In a coauthored paper from 2013, "The Genetic Basis for Elite Running Performance," he pointed to another study that says "the heritability of athlete status is 66 percent." More broadly, he and his fellow authors conclude that just because one or two "candidate genes" do not hold the key to a genetic explanation of Kenyan running success, it does not mean there is no genetic answer. The human genome is complex. Around two hundred gene variants, Tucker noted, have so far been associated with physical fitness and athleticism.

Tucker is sensitive to the fact that genome-wide studies are still in their infancy. He argues that it is stiflingly complex to distinguish between genetic makeup (what you might call innate ability) and a panoply of nongenetic factors such as diet, the intensity of training, the desire to achieve, and so on.

As far as explaining the Kenyan running phenomenon, all of these arguments seem to point to a dark forest of the unknown. We do, however, already understand many things about how athletic talent manifests itself in the genes. For instance, as Tucker points out, there has been impressive research to pinpoint how "trainable" a person is—that is, how quickly and effectively he or she responds to training. Dr. Claude Bouchard of the Huffines Institute for Sports Medicine & Human Performance in Texas has pinpointed 21 single nucleotide polymorphisms (or SNPs) out of a panel of 325,000 in the human genome that account for about half of one's VO_2 max response to aerobic training. That is to say, we can tell from a genetic study which person will get fitter, quicker, than another. "High responders" have 19 or more of these SNPs; "low responders" have 9 or fewer. (High responders obviously have a much greater chance of becoming professional athletes.)

There has been no large study of the Kalenjin population to see what percentage are high responders to training. But from the anecdotal evidence, the number of highly trainable men and women in the Kalenjin population seems remarkable. People seem to walk off the farms and into training groups. Somehow, in a couple of years, they're competing in big races. One only needs to hear a few of these tales to wonder whether there isn't something heritable in the sheer speed at which no-hopers are transformed into champions.

John Manners, an American scientist and historian of road running who has spent many years in Kenya, told one great story about a young and rather fat Kalenjin named Paul Rotich. In 1988, when Rotich was twenty-two years old, his father, an affluent farmer, sent him to South Plains College, in Texas, with $10,000 to pay for his room and board. The money was meant to last two years, but Rotich spent almost all of it by the end of his first year. If he was to stay in college, he needed to find another source of income.

Rotich considered his options. There were other Kalenjin men at his college who were supported by track scholarships. Although he was a dumpy five foot eight and 189 pounds, and had never raced competitively in his life, he started to train. He was so ashamed of his physique that he ran on the track at night, but he quickly lost weight and gained speed. By the fall, he made the cross-country team. He then finished in the top fifty in the National Junior College Championships, went on to win a track scholarship to Lubbock Christian University, and earned all-American honors ten times in cross-country and track. Upon Rotich's return to Kenya, his cousin said: "So it is true. If you can run, any Kalenjin can run."

——

There may be a more obvious factor that helps explain why Kalen-jins are better at long-distance running than everybody else. It's sometimes omitted from arguments about the dominance of Kenya because it seems to be a racial stereotype, one that belongs in the fieldbook of some nineteenth-century English colonialist. But one can't help noticing that, with some exceptions, Kalenjins *look* like they should be good at running long distances. To use the language of geneticists, you'd say the Kalenjin runner's "phe-notype" was perfect for marathons, with a short body and, as has been mentioned before, those long, slender, birdlike legs.

Naturally, not every Kalenjin looks like this. They have their share of fat guys and plump matrons. But there may just be a higher proportion of people in this population with a good phe-notype for running. And since running is such a big deal in this part of the world, pretty much all of them give the sport a try. The chances of converting talent into elite-level success, there-fore, are high.

East Africa, however, does not have a monopoly on such "talent." People with the potential for distance running success exist in other populations, albeit in slightly weaker concentra-tions. Mike Joyner, for one, is convinced that America has its own marathon stars in waiting. It's possible they are swept up by other sports, don't know the path to distance running success, or are unwilling to break themselves training for a sport with little obvious financial reward. But these kids exist if we only know where to look for them.

Joyner believes there is one significant untapped resource in America: Native Americans from the Four Corners region of southwest America. To make his point, he tells a story about running against a Native American named Al Waquie in the late 1970s. Waquie was from the Walatowa Pueblo of Jemez tribe. Joyner raced against him at the La Luz trail race at Sandia Peak in Albuquerque, New Mexico. Waquie won in some style, beating Ric Rojas, one of the top-ranked distance runners in America at the time, by between two and three minutes in a race lasting an hour or so. This was just one exceptional performance among many. Joyner believes that Waquie was the "best runner you've never heard of."

Joyner also points out that Waquie's exploits are part of a wider story of running talent from Native American communities in the Four Corners. Like the Kalenjin and the Oromo, the Navajo and Hopi communities have spent significant time at altitude. Their cultures also prize running ability. But unlike in East Africa, there has been no outpouring of elite running talent from this part of the world. Perhaps the most famous Hopi runner was Lewis Tewanima, who won a silver medal at the Stockholm Olympics in 1912 at 10,000m and set a U.S. record that was not surpassed for a half century. Since then, it's been slim pickings.

Cross-country is still a big sport in the Four Corners. Every year, there is a large meeting in which Navajo and Hopi competitors "Race the Rez" (the reservation). Tuba City High School, in Arizona, wins state championship after state championship. But for many reasons, including but not limited to a seeming unwillingness on the part of promising Native American juniors to turn professional and leave their home district, this wellspring of talent does not progress to the elite level.

—

As the shoe designers know, there is something particular and measurable about the Kalenjins that makes them an interesting study group in this debate. As a group, they carry less distal weight on their legs, so it requires less energy for them to move at 2:05 pace than it would for a European runner with chunkier ankles.

This trait might seem to point to an obvious genetic advantage the Kenyans possess. And, in one sense, that's true. But there's a complicating factor in the debate about bodyshapes, because running success comes in many forms. Yes, Kalenjin athletes are generally skinny, stringy guys. And yes, lighter, thinner lower legs seem to be important in distance running success. But look at the range of bodyshapes of men who win long races and you see a surprisingly various group.

Some Kalenjin runners, like Philemon Rono, are almost childishly tiny; some, such as the bullish Geoffrey Kamworor, are built more powerfully, like 800m runners. Meanwhile, many of the greatest runners from other parts of East Africa are constructed from an entirely different instruction manual. Sammy Wanjiru, a Kikuyu, was short and—in relative terms—powerfully built, with a sprinter's thighs. His old Ethiopian rival Tsegaye Kebede, who won the Chicago Marathon in 2012 and the London Marathon in 2013, is five foot nothing and runs like a windup toy. Haile's body looks nothing like Wilson Kipsang's.

All marathon champions share one characteristic: they are whippet thin. This makes sense. The more weight one carries, the more energy one expends carrying it. Over two hours, these fractions add up. But what about the more complicated question of the shape of someone's frame allowing them to run faster? If the bodyshape of runners is the key to their efficiency—how much energy it takes to propel them along the road—then there appear to be many efficient bodyshapes.

How do these observations relate back to genetics? At present, geneticists struggle to pinpoint exactly to what degree one's height is inherited from one's parents. Determining the genetic basis of height would seem to be relatively simple. But even this trait appears to be the product of the interplay between one's DNA—the instruction manual—and the environment into which one is born.

In Japan, to use one dramatic example, the average height of eleven-year-old boys increased by 5½ inches between 1951 and 2001. If height were purely determined by our DNA, such wild statistical improvements would not be possible. Clearly, there is something else going on when the numbers shift so violently.

Take the aspect of genetics we're now trying to understand— that of outlier athletic ability. Is it possible to pinpoint exactly which parts of our DNA are useful, or essential, to becoming an elite runner? In 2008, Alun Williams, of Manchester Metropolitan University in England, identified twenty-three genes associated to a greater or lesser degree with success in endurance events. But he and his team calculated that the chances of a person being born with all the "right" versions of these genes was one in a quadrillion (one thousand million million). Nobody on earth, he estimated, was a genetically perfect endurance athlete. One could only be less imperfect.

———

What's been most interesting about the recent developments in genomics, the science of how genes relate to one another, is the reemergence of the idea that environments may determine how our genes are *expressed*. Denis Noble, a biologist and philosopher from Oxford University, uses a beautiful metaphor to explain this idea: "the Music of Life." He likes to think of our genetic code as a musical instrument rather than a set of instructions to be followed to the letter. Genes, he says, are not a "blueprint for life" but rather, because they work in systems and groups, more like a set of organ pipes that can be played.

To reduce the particulars of this nuanced theory to a basic level, Noble rejects the idea of genes determining our lives. DNA, he argues, is not a "read-only" file. He argues that not only is information fed from our genes upward, but our bodies also receive information from the world around them and feed that information back "downward."

Our DNA, meanwhile, is not the only means by which traits are passed from one generation to another. There is increasing evidence that, through our maternal lines, the behavior of our parents and ancestors can influence ways in which our genes are turned "off" or "on." This study of non-DNA inheritance is part of the growing field of epigenetics. If it's true that our development is influenced not only by the mixture of our genetic makeup and our environment, but also by the lifestyle choices of our parents, then we might understand the dominance of the high-living, hardworking Kalenjin a little better.

John Manners, the American Kenyaphile who told the story of the roly-poly Paul Rotich and his subsequent athletic success, posited a tentative and controversial theory about the development of Kalenjin running. He argued that not only are the Kalenjin pastoralists, leading active, outdoor lifestyles, but they have traditionally practiced cattle raiding—or theft, to be less polite. In the past, these raids could take the form of treks as long as 100 miles. And there was a prize for being successful.

In his paper "Kenya's Running Tribe," Manners suggested, "The better a young man was at raiding—in large part, a function of his speed and endurance—the more cattle he accumulated. And since cattle were what a prospective husband needed to pay for a bride, the more a young man had, the more wives he could buy, and the more children he was likely to father. It is not hard to imagine that such a reproductive advantage might cause a significant shift in a group's genetic makeup over the course of a few centuries."

When the British ruled in Kenya, they attempted to stamp out the practice of cattle raiding. According to one history of the region, athletic meetings were organized in the late 1930s by the colonial authorities so that Kalenjin men could show their "valor in sports and games, not war." Manners also observed that the "austere warrior culture" and the brutal Kalenjin circumcision ceremonies, which still exist today, might have bred toughness.

It's difficult to know what to make of this. The cattle-raiding hypothesis is intriguing but unprovable. And although the Kalenjin runners I have met are tough, their trade demands that they be so. Professional marathoners are a hardy breed. But the cattle-raiding idea seems to tally with what we are now starting to understand about how the lifestyles of our parents affects the expression of our DNA. Long-distance running has been culturally important to the Kalenjin. It would be strange to think that this facet of their history is not instrumental in them trouncing all comers at the marathon.

The work of Denis Noble bathes the African champions in a new light. Of the hundreds and thousands of men and women in Ethiopia and Kenya who attempt to have careers as professional runners, these particular athletes play the music of their lives most sweetly. Their success is always built on the necessary foundations of the high, active childhood, the good bodyshape, willing muscles, Spartan work ethic, and some ultimately unknowable conversation between their past and their present. But genes, and heritage, only explain so much. Certain, special athletes need to be champions, and will work themselves half to death for the success they crave.

——

The elephant sitting in the corner of this debating chamber is the matter of drugs. Dope infects almost all professional sports. For every athlete who wishes to ascend to the highest plane of competition under his own steam, there will always be athletes who desire a shortcut. Marathon running is no different. Dopers have prospered from the beginning. Tom Hicks won the St. Louis Olympic marathon jacked up on strychnine and brandy, and it nearly killed him. That was in 1904.

There was once an Elysian view of the sport of distance running that willfully exempted East Africans from the temptations of others. Journalists saw the humble manner in which Kenyan and Ethiopian runners lived and concluded that cheating in such circumstances simply wasn't possible. East Africans, it was thought, possessed neither the know-how nor the iceboxes to dope. For a time there was a thin joke in marathon circles that the only substance victorious Kenyans were likely to test positive for was *ugali*.

This myth has now been exploded. In the past two years, several East African distance runners have tested positive for performance-enhancing drugs, including steroids and the hormone erythropoietin, or EPO, which stimulates red-blood-cell production and therefore the transport of oxygen in the bloodstream. In 2012, an investigation by the German television channel ARD also claimed to have found evidence of blood transfusions and human growth hormone (HGH) in Kenyan running country.

Some of the busted athletes have been well-known figures, but the majority have been nobodies. Kenyans have tested positive in greater numbers than Ethiopians, although this fact alone doesn't tell us whether there is a greater or lesser problem in either country—it only means there have been more positive tests in Kenya. What we know is that if there ever was a blissful period in which nobody from East Africa possessed the inclination or the means to dope, it is now over.

The question everybody with an interest in the sport would like to know the answer to is this: how big is the problem? Should we suspect every great Kenyan or Ethiopian marathon performance? There are no simple answers, and no simple means to advance one's understanding. In Kenya, where most of the biggest doping stories broke in 2012 and 2013, and where the exploits of the country's runners are an issue not only of national pride but of profound economic significance, the issue became contentious and fiercely politicized. Foreign journalists asking difficult questions risked exclusion from the country.

The athletes, however, talked about it plenty among themselves. In recent years, as the money has risen in road racing, and the times for the marathon have dropped, running country has been awash with innuendo. The rumor mill is laughably inconsistent. One day a piece of gossip will reach you that so-and-so is *definitely* up to something. The next day someone else tells you that the same so-and-so is as honest as the day is long. One is always grateful for these vacillating narratives because they are a reminder not to believe everything people tell you on this matter.

In Kenya, doping accusations are sharpened like *pangas*. A journeyman runner looks at a champion who has just run 2:03 to win a major marathon, and whispers *huyo amemeza dawa:* "that one is on drugs." The champion looks at a journeyman who has just run a personal best of 2:09, winning a race in China with lax doping controls, and hisses the same thing.

Chapter Eight

Only with Blood

THE WEATHER was foul outside, and in the twin room of the
four-star hotel in which they were staying, two low-level Kenyan runners prepared their vests and bibs for the following day's
marathon. They wanted to talk to me about drugs, and spoke
on condition of anonymity. Their personal bests were relatively
modest in Kenyan terms, and they barely covered their expenses
to travel to a race in a bleak European capital with only a few
thousand euros in prize money. They talked for a long time as
they sat on their beds, with the burble of the television and the
sound of rain against the windows in the background.

The two runners said that, in Kenya, there were "so many
bad doctors you can't count them." They described a system
whereby these "doctors," who were mostly quack pharmacists
based in the town of Eldoret, would sell an athlete a course of
performance-enhancing drugs in exchange either for cash or a
share of his winnings. The drug in question, although they didn't
name it explicitly, seemed to be EPO. (They referred often to a

drug for "the blood.") And the relationship between the athlete and the "doctor," said the two runners, was "twenty-four/seven." They were always on hand to provide masking agents should the testers come calling.

Most of this information was talked about openly enough, especially among European agents and coaches (although before my meeting with the two low-level athletes, I had never heard such a detailed description of the process). Some Kenyan stars also discussed the problem in a roundabout way. In the narratives of many high-profile athletes, doping was seen as something that "lazy" runners did in lieu of training. This was a willfully wrongheaded view. As the Tour de France scandals showed, drugs are used for precisely the opposite reason: to train and race *harder*. Moreover, doping was always, in the opinion of the bigger names, a problem that affected the underclass of the sport, because inferior athletes lacked the "natural" talent. (Even Brother Colm O'Connell shared this view. He told an Irish newspaper that doping was generally used by "mediocre" athletes, looking for an "edge.")

The two athletes in the hotel room reversed this equation. They named almost every star in Kenyan marathon running and accused them of doping.

The allegations were shocking, but both runners were markedly short on proof of any kind, and the basis for their specific charges against individual runners seemed thin. The athlete-whistleblowers trained in Iten, alongside hundreds of others, and their stories were drawn from a mixture of rumor and common-sense calculation. They knew of the existence of the pharmacies and the "doctors." And they simply didn't believe it was possible to run the spectacular times that had now become commonplace on the marathon circuit without illegal assistance. These two runners, who had personal bests above 2:10, said anything below 2:06 for a marathon was "suspicious."

One of the runners laughed when I expressed surprise.

"You think you can run two-oh-three, only with *blood*?" he asked.

Well, yes—I did think that.

———

Take a step back. From a layman's perspective, it's not obvious what kind of edge EPO would give a Kenyan who has already spent his whole life running at altitude. The number of red blood cells in his system is already likely to be high, and there is a limit to how many red blood cells a person can have before he is at risk of a heart attack or stroke. (This dangerous abundance of red blood cells is known in medicine as polycythemia.)

But this apparent common sense is wrong. EPO *does* help altitude-born-and-raised Kenyans. A recent study by the University of Glasgow conducted tests on a group of Scottish runners, and on Kenyan athletes from running country, and found their performances both benefited equally from a course of EPO. It's ridiculous to suggest, as the coach Renato Canova once claimed in an online debate, that blood manipulation would have no effect on top Kenyan athletes. Who knows how a marathoner might use EPO? In the Tour de France, the hormone was often used as a kind of recuperation aid.

If there were a wonder drug for distance runners, it would be one that aided recovery. Marathoners have always logged extraordinary mileage, and their biggest problem is staying healthy for races. Derek Clayton, the tall Australian who broke the world record twice in the late 1960s, sometimes ran 200 miles a week in training. Partly as a result of his debilitating work ethic, he was prone to injuries.

Few of today's marathoners run so far, but their training schedules are if anything more destructive than Clayton's. The "high volume, high intensity" philosophy requires a mixture of speedwork sessions lasting an hour or more in order to build resistance to a fast race pace, and long runs at a high tempo. Being able to complete such punishing sessions day after day is the key to staying competitive in the marathon. So it is in the field of recovery that the marathon is most vulnerable to cheating. In theory, athletes could stop taking illicit substances weeks before a race, and show up to a marathon clean—with hundreds of high quality, ill-gotten miles in their legs.

But not many Kenyans have actually been caught with EPO. Curiously, most have been busted for steroids. The most shocking case of recent years involved a Kenyan runner named Mathew Kisorio. He tested positive for a banned anabolic steroid, norandrosterone, at the national championships in June 2012. Looking back, Kisorio's story told us much about the shape and size of the Kenyan doping issue, not least because, for a short time after he was popped, he talked freely.

———

Kisorio's failed test was particularly surprising to me. He was one of the first elite Kenyans I watched in training, and I knew his coach—Claudio Berardelli—as well as anybody involved in the elite marathon. I'd often stayed at Berardelli's house in Eldoret, eaten his pasta, and listened to his entertainingly opinionated views on the sport. His polemics were punctuated both by curious English translations of Italian phrases (Berardelli said "touch my balls" when an English person would say "cross my fingers") and by the constant ringing of his phone. Often it was an athlete on the other end of the line who had found himself in some scrape or another.

In all this time, Berardelli seemed honest, industrious, and virulently antidoping. Part of the reason he was involved in distance running, he said, was that he had become disillusioned with cycling. He was once a promising junior rider in Italy but abandoned the sport when his contemporaries became involved in blood manipulation and other dirty tricks.

When the news broke of Kisorio's bust, it was natural that Berardelli would be the subject of suspicion. Not only was he the athlete's coach, but he was from northern Italy, an area that had been at the nexus of recent doping scandals in Europe. (Lance Armstrong's doctor and doping enabler, Dr. Michele Ferrari, was from the region.) If you saw only these basic facts, there was an easy narrative around Kisorio. an Italian Svengali, frustrated by recent results, juiced up his star athlete using "European" methods. But the scattershot evidence that emerged after Kisorio's failed test told a different, and much more Kenyan, story.

I first met Kisorio in June 2011, almost exactly a year before he failed the drug test. A tall athlete with an intense mien and a pleasingly uninhibited running style, he was hoping to move from the track to the roads. No doubt, Kisorio was a talent. He won a silver in the World Junior Championships at 5,000m and had recorded impressive personal bests for both the 5,000m and 10,000m. But he was beset by a weakness in his kick. Often, Kisorio would be in contention with a lap to go, only to find himself outsprinted, finishing in sixth or seventh place, and earning lousy money. Because of his struggles on the track, Kisorio decided to move to the roads, where a lack of kick was not such a problematic fault.

On the day we met, Kisorio was training on dirt roads around a tea plantation in Nandi. Berardelli drove behind Kisorio and his training partners in a pickup truck. One by one, Kisorio's fellow runners jumped into the back of the truck, winded and unable to live with the pace. By the end of the two-hour session, Kisorio ran on his own, knocking out the final miles in a destructively fast cadence—his eyes fixed as if in a trance, and sweat glimmering on his high cheekbones. At the time, it was the most impressive training run I had ever witnessed.

Some months later, at the Philadelphia half marathon, Kisorio made good on this bedrock of preparation when he won the race in 58 minutes and 46 seconds. His time was both a new American all-comers record and the fourth-fastest half marathon ever recorded. Five years earlier, it would have been a world record. Any way you looked at the performance, it seemed to announce the arrival of a significant new road-running star.

But Kisorio struggled at the full marathon distance. He was in contention on debut at the 2011 New York Marathon, in the same race that Geoffrey Mutai slaughtered the course record, before fading badly in the final miles. In Boston, the next year, he endured the same problem. In hot weather, he ran a fast midpart of the race and was leading at 30km but imploded before the final section and finished tenth.

He returned to Kenya dejected. This is when—according to his own testimony, and a discussion he had with Berardelli after his doping bust—he decided to visit a shady "doctor" in Eldoret. Before Boston, it seems, Kisorio was clean.

Not much is known about Kisorio's visit to the "doctor" except that it was in Eldoret, and that the athlete didn't ask too many questions. Kisorio told Hajo Seppelt, a German investigative reporter from the television channel ARD, that he complained to the doctor about a "power of endurance" problem. This doctor, whose identity has not been revealed, reassured Kisorio that he would "take care of it." The athlete said he was given tablets. Seppelt also reported that Kisorio spoke of "injections" of a substance that the German journalist took to mean EPO.

Berardelli has questioned this aspect of Kisorio's testimony. After the athlete's failed test, Berardelli says he was profoundly shocked and hurt, and, against the advice of some, sought a meeting with Kisorio. At that meeting, it became clear to Berardelli not only that Kisorio had intended to cheat but that he possessed only the faintest idea of what EPO actually was. Kisorio told Berardelli that the doctor had conducted some initial tests on his blood profile, and told him that he "didn't have enough blood." He suggested a course of injections to improve his "volume."

But when Kisorio tested positive some weeks later, it was not for EPO but for a banned steroid—norandrosterone. Are we to assume this is what he was injecting? The athlete clearly had no idea. Norandrosterone is an analogue of testosterone. It can be used to quicken muscle repair and to create more red cells in the blood, and is sometimes used in medicine as an anemia treatment. What makes norandrosterone a puzzling drug to take as a doper is that it is so easy to detect. It stays in an athlete's system for months.

Kisorio knew what he was doing was wrong, even if he had no idea about what he was taking, or about the risks of detection. When he was scheduled for the test at the national championships, he called the pharmacy to see whether his sample would show up clean. The doctor told him there was no problem, and Kisorio happily trotted over to the antidoping tent to give a urine sample. When the test came back positive, Kisorio called the doctor again, enraged. "Yes," said the doctor, "you should probably have waited a few days."

Having been busted, Kisorio was furious with the doctor. He started burning bridges. In an interview with the German reporter, Kisorio said that doping was "widespread" among Kenyan athletes, and that his doctor had showed him a list of other runners assisted by the same doping program. (Again, he failed to share the names on the list, if indeed it existed.)

In any event, Berardelli swears he knew nothing of Kisorio's doping program and suggests that another athlete introduced him to the doctor. One's natural reaction to such a statement would be disbelief. How, you might wonder, could a coach *not* know his athlete was doping? In other sports, in other countries, such a situation would be utterly implausible. But in Kenya there is a high degree of autonomy on the part of athletes—even those who employ coaches. Kisorio's own testimony indicated that his management team was not involved with his decision to dope. Having stayed with Berardelli for long periods, witnessed how his athletes live, and reported on several Kenyan doping cases, this scenario rings true to me.

What Kisorio's story seemed to demonstrate was that it was possible for Kenyan athletes to access illegal drugs in a way that largely excluded *muzungus*. This is not to say that foreign managers are blameless. There are, no doubt, some who have introduced athletes to drugs (the names of *muzungu* and Kenyan facilitators have been mentioned to me, but I have seen no proof of their involvement, and do not intend to libel them here). There may also be a wider problem of deliberate blindness on the part of "clean" foreign managers who put their fingers in their ears and whistle while their athletes get up to who knows what, and then collect their percentage of winnings. In either case, it seems the dirty work is largely left up to the runners themselves.

———

The most illuminating interventions in the Kenyan doping scandals were those made by the sports politicians. After Kisorio's claim that cheating was "widespread" in Kenya, Isaiah Kiplagat, the chairman of Athletics Kenya, responded by saying that Kisorio was the only Kenyan doper he knew of—and therefore, it was suggested, a bad apple in an otherwise pristine barrel. Kiplagat then demanded that all foreign coaches without work permits leave the country immediately.

In October 2012, after the German journalist Hajo Seppelt's documentary on Kenyan doping, Kiplagat delivered a wide-ranging jeremiad to local journalists. He said that foreign coaches were "behind all these claims and their aim is to portray Kenyan athletes in bad light in the pretext of coaching them. These coaches have been extracting blood from some athletes and mixing them with other things to qualify their doping claims. They are even responsible for calling in international journalists and feeding them with their doping lies. They also house the same international journalists in their apartments when they come from abroad in a bid to sell their malicious doping campaigns better.

"Kenyans generally work hard," Kiplagat continued. "It's not possible to beat Kenyans who train even ten times a day as compared to other foreign athletes who train once a day. Kenyans are about hard work and other people should not try to twist things to justify their failures. We have nothing to do with drugs, we simply work hard. For the doubting Thomases, you can look at Kenya's athletic performance since the 1960s before making malicious conclusions."

The reality, as Kiplagat must have known, was rather different. Several doping cases pointed to the existence of pharmacies in Eldoret, and at least one in the capital, Nairobi, where illicit drugs were said to be available to athletes. But instead of targeting the apparent source of the problem—the pharmacies—Athletics Kenya chose to throw around wild accusations. In public at least, both Athletics Kenya and the police seemed to view the existence of such outlets phlegmatically.

When Wilson Loyanae Erupe, a marathoner from Turkana, in northern Kenya, was busted for EPO in 2013, several sources say he gave up the name of his Eldoret pharmacist to Athletics Kenya. Before he was caught, Loyanae had enjoyed an incredible few months, in both senses of the word. The high point of his 2012 season was winning the Seoul Marathon in 2:05:37, shaving four minutes from his personal best.

When he was caught cheating months later, he offered up the name of his "doctor." This might have been the moment to smash a doping ring. But Kenyan politics demanded a different solution. Although I learned that the pharmacist in question was quietly put out of business, his client list was not exposed, and no further progress in rooting out drugs cheats has been made. The Kenyan media, meanwhile, did not press Athletics Kenya on this matter. Is it possible Loyanae was the only runner to visit this shady pharmacist?

These "doctors" can make serious money. From anecdotal evidence gathered in 2012 and 2013, the price for a course of EPO ranged from 65,000 Kenyan shillings (around $750) to 100,000 KES (around $1,150). Often, runners didn't have the money up front, so the cost of treatment was recouped as a percentage of future winnings, meaning that some middle-ranking athletes entered into an irreversible relationship with their dealers. Who knows what they were buying? Some of the treatments, I was told, were "Chinese," some were fake, and some were stolen from the Moi Teaching Hospital in Eldoret, which uses EPO in its renal and intensive care units. (A visiting physician at the hospital confirmed that there had been thefts from the hospital stores.)

This was all dispiriting information. But if this was a Kenyan "system," it was one marked by a distinct lack of sophistication, and a far cry from the intricate maneuvering described by whistle-blowers in Tour de France doping cases. In its reasoned decision against the cyclist Lance Armstrong in 2013, for instance, the United States Anti-Doping Agency described a highly professional doping system that had kept Armstrong and his team of riders chemically ahead of his competitors for years. There were couriers who delivered drugs by moped under cover of darkness, doctors who monitored the blood levels of riders on a constant basis, and handlers who possessed detailed knowledge of when a rider would be vulnerable to testing. There were also millions of dollars in backhand payments.

Now, look at the most high-profile Kenyan drugs case. Kisorio is nobody's idea of an evil genius. He appears to be confused about what, exactly, he put in his own body. So, on the one hand, the stories of men like Kisorio are cause for serious concern for anybody with a love for the marathon. But on the other, there is little evidence that the cheating has been professionalized, in the manner of cycling's worst years.

As Coach Patrick Sang told me, the situation in Kenya was not so endemic it could not be cured. "I was a top-level athlete for seventeen years, and I know it's possible to compete at the highest level without cheating," he said. "I also know there is a problem. But all you need to do is to criminalize it. It's not just a question of bans from the sport. Make it a matter for the police."

———

Perhaps it is naïve to believe that drugs did not become endemic in distance running long ago. There are experienced people in the sport who believe that the elite have been doping for years. Those views come from surprising places. In 1999, for instance, Mo Farah's coach, Alberto Salazar, gave a presentation to the Duke Conference on Doping in Sport, in which he made several fascinating remarks, not least this one: "I believe that it is currently difficult to be among the top five in the world in any of the distance events without using EPO or Human Growth Hormone. While some of the top athletes may be clean, so many athletes are running so fast that their performances are suspect. This is compounded for me by the fact that the times these athletes are running just happen to coincide exactly with what top exercise physiologists have calculated taking EPO would produce."

In 1999, there could be no doubt about the top two distance runners in the world: Haile Gebrselassie of Ethiopia and Paul Tergat of Kenya. Was Salazar saying that he believed these athletes were dopers? (Salazar says he no longer stands by the comments he made in 1999, and that he "did not reference the athletes you call out.")

A decade and a half after making his remarks, Salazar was coach to undoubtedly the top distance runner on the track in the world: Mo Farah. The coach is also the subject of scrutiny about his methods. In 2013, a long investigation in the *Wall Street Journal* of Salazar and Nike's relationship with a doctor named Jeffrey Brown found that many of Salazar's athletes had been treated by Brown for a syndrome called "hypothyroidism." Galen Rupp was one such patient. Treating athletes for hypothyroidism is not illegal, and it's also not clear what kind of benefit it would give an elite runner. But the very fact that so many of Salazar's charges have been diagnosed with the condition has caused suspicion. After Jos Hermens of Global Sports watched his athletes being trounced at the 2012 London Olympics by Salazar's athletes, he told a Dutch journalist, "Science has triumphed over nature."

As for the supposedly "widespread" nature of doping in East Africa, Frank Shorter, America's last Olympic champion at the marathon distance, had his suspicions even before the most recent busts. He believed that Kenyan dominance in the sport was catalyzed by doping in the 1990s. In 2011, Shorter gave this devastating précis of the professional marathon running era to *Runner's World* magazine: "Once it became apparent that a Kenyan could come over here and in two years make enough to purchase a farm and become the patriarch of an extended family, that really is what produced the Rift Valley running explosion. Those Kenyans then moved to foreign countries, got coaches and agents, who in many cases were doctors, and the drug thing entered. I always said, put a Kenyan on drugs and it's all over. Let's be realistic—that happened."

———

Should we consider every fast marathon as suspicious? It seems like an unwarranted and cynical view. And anyway, what counts as suspicious? 2:06? 2:04? 2:02? In his paper on the possibility of the two-hour marathon, Mike Joyner estimated a physiological ceiling for running a marathon: the startlingly precise time of 1:57:58. So what extra time on top of that 1:57:58 should we allow our best runners?

Joyner is somewhat at a loss. EPO and blood transfusion techniques entered cycling in earnest in the 1990s, and he believes it is naïve to think they didn't enter running to some degree as well. As a result, it's hard for him to project what a reasonable time for the marathon is, because he doesn't know who in the past ran clean and who ran dirty. All statistics in this area are corrupted to some degree—it's just a question of how badly.

What we do know is that in order for the sport of professional marathon running to have a viable future, testing needs to become more thorough. At the time of writing, there was no permanent blood-testing facility in either Kenya or Ethiopia to monitor athletes year-round. In order for a blood sample from East Africa to be tested, it was necessary to put it on at least two flights to reach a laboratory in Geneva. (The plan was for a World Anti-Doping Agency–approved facility to be completed in Kenya by the end of 2014; the London Marathon contributed funds to the WADA project.)

Without regular out-of-season blood tests, cheats will have slipped through the net. There is urine testing, on an ad hoc basis, there is blood testing at big races, and there are now "biological passports" carried by top athletes, which should catch discrepancies between readings given at different events. But the system was not as comprehensive as it should have been.

Moreover, there was a large political aspect to the problem. In 2013, the Canadian lawyer Dick Pound wrote a report for WADA in which he bemoaned the unwillingness of certain countries to catch dopers. After the report was published, a WADA representative told me he was "aghast" at the situation in Kenya. The WADA agent believed that the doping controls in the country were haphazard, and that the national athletics federation had not been open about its efforts to stamp out the problem. If this assessment was true, you could see why it might be so. If the Kenyan authorities were to expose running country to heat and light, they might see things they wish they had not seen.

With accusation and rumor swirling around Kenya's marathon stars, most athletes talked only in vague, general terms about the problem. But Geoffrey Mutai was happy to speak up. His name had been mentioned in conversations about drugs. That in itself was not unusual. If you listened to running country gossip for long enough, you'd hear every single Kenyan champion sullied by innuendo. Mutai fell under more suspicion than most not only because had he run fantastic times in an aggressive manner, but because he was said to have been friendly with Kisorio, the most notorious Kenyan doper, before his bust.

(I reinforce the point about such stories in Kenya. I treated these rumors as rumors. In the three years I reported on Mutai, he was tested many times for blood and urine. He has never given a positive test. What's more, there was never a scrap of circumstantial evidence to suggest he had ever doped. An IAAF tester working in Kenya also confirmed he had no suspicions about Mutai.)

Mutai knew the gossip and addressed it directly. He utterly rejected the claim that he had ever cheated, and the more incendiary claim that he had introduced Kisorio to the pharmacy where he was treated for his "power of endurance" problem. He said that he wanted more testing more often to prove his innocence.

"I am clean," he said. "I want all athletes in Kenya to remain clean. Anytime, anywhere, I am ready for testing. It gives me pain when people see me run fast and say I have used drugs. If I have used them, then God take everything from me, I cannot enjoy it."

On the subject of the dodgy "doctors" in Eldoret, however, he offered an interesting perspective. He said that it was sometimes the case that athletes really didn't know what they were putting in their bodies, but that this was not an excuse. Part of what a "doctor" offered an athlete was plausible deniability. Mutai said Kisorio was attempting to cheat even if he didn't know what drug he was taking. It was easy to say that you had visited your doctor, and he had given you something you didn't understand, and it had shown up in a positive test. In Mutai's opinion, this problem could be solved if the Kenyan authorities built a hospital in Eldoret only for athletes. Then "nobody could explain, 'Oh, I went to the doctor and he gave me this medicine.' "

Geoffrey Mutai was one of those athletes upon whom suspicion would always rest. In his major marathon career, he had transformed what people believed possible in the sport. But his success, tragically, came at a cost to his reputation. Unless more is done to enforce WADA guidelines, any runner who follows in his rapid footsteps will face the same problem. You can be sure that if and when a man breaks two hours for the marathon, the whiff of disbelief will hang around him every day of his life.

Chapter Nine

He Kills Everybody

April and September 2013

THE DAY that broke in London on the morning of Sunday, April 21, 2013, was like a gift from the marathon gods. The temperature was in the low forties, the sun shone weakly, and there was not a cloud in the sky. In the early morning, the lobby of London's Guoman Tower Hotel, a lumpen concrete building that sits on the banks of the River Thames in the shadow of Tower Bridge, vibrated with chatter. A handful of the most accomplished marathon runners on the planet had been assembled for the season's most prestigious road race on a morning designed for speed. Waiting for the double-decker bus to leave for the startline, Geoffrey Mutai leaned on the back of a chair, staring out from beneath his Adidas hoodie, with his arms folded in front of him. He tapped one foot, and an impish smile spread across his face. He was not the only runner feeling skittish.

It wasn't just the lineup, or the conditions, that prompted this nervous energy. London always has a stacked field, and it hums on marathon day, whatever the weather. Since the first race was run in 1981, the city, normally so phlegmatic, is forced into a goofy grin. The event is cynicism-proof. But the atmosphere on the morning of the 2013 London Marathon was unique: a combination of a deep, defiant joy, and a palpable tension. Six days earlier, two brothers named Tamerlan and Dzhokhar Tsarnaev had detonated pressure-cooker bombs at the finish line of the Boston Marathon, killing three people and wounding more than two hundred others.

There was something particularly calculated about the attack on the finish line in Boston. Its evil lay not only in the sudden and shocking reversal of a life-affirming festival into a howling crime scene, but because it reminded everyone of the vulnerability of a city marathon. Too many people are involved in a race, over too long a distance, for every security angle to be covered. Part of the joy of the marathon is the fact that supporters crowd the barriers to shout for their loved ones; that, for a few hours, the race and the city embrace one another. What the Tsarnaev brothers did was to attack the very idea of that openness. It seemed obvious, too, that the marathon was an attractive target for the terrorists because of the rolling media coverage at the finish line. The Tsarnaevs didn't need to wait for the television trucks to arrive. The cameras were already there.

The Boston Marathon was held, as always, on a Monday, only six days before the race in London. Four days after the bombs went off, and two days before London, a manhunt was still under way for one of the terrorists, and the city of Boston was on lockdown. During this tense period, there was widespread confusion as to why the event had been targeted in the first place. It would have been easy, in the light of such concerns, to cancel the London Marathon. Instead, the organizers decided that life, and the race, must go on.

———

In purely sporting terms, the race already contained all the ingredients for drama. The men's field was perhaps the most distinguished ever assembled. It included the world record holder (Patrick Makau), the current London champion (Wilson Kipsang), the reigning Chicago champion and former London champion (Tsegaye Kebede), two former London champions (Emmanuel Mutai and Martin Lel), and the Olympic champion (Stephen Kiprotich of Uganda), in addition to a host of other studs: Feyisa Lilesa and Ayele Abshero of Ethiopia, and Stanley Biwott of Kenya. There was also excitement at the prospect of watching Mo Farah, Britain's 5,000m and 10,000m Olympic gold medalist and the new darling of distance running, complete the first half of the marathon in preparation for his full-marathon debut the following year.

And then there was Geoffrey Mutai. Nobody knew quite what to expect from him. After 2011, the year in which he remade the sport, his racing life had not been so smooth. In his first marathon of 2012, in Boston, Mutai failed to finish in soaring temperatures, complaining of stomach cramps. Although many strong runners were affected by the heat, whispers began to circulate that Mutai was not the same athlete who performed wonders the previous year. There was loose talk in Kenya of drinking, of complacency, of overtraining, of undertraining. Because of his inability to complete Boston, Mutai was left out of Kenya's marathon team for the London Olympics—a team that also traveled without Patrick Makau, the world record holder. Mutai discovered his omission from the Olympic squad when he turned on the television news one night.

Mutai had formed a plan to silence the doubters in Berlin 2012, but it came unstuck for a variety of reasons, including the frozen pace car and the slight injury he carried with him to Germany from the muddy tracks of Skyland. Although his 2:04:15 in Berlin was the fastest time of 2012, and although he had run those startling course records in Boston and New York only months earlier, one highly regarded coach gave this brutal assessment: "Maybe the Geoffrey of 2011 is finished. In Kenya they come and then . . ." The coach made a swooping motion with his hand, like a crashing airplane.

Mutai disregarded the talk. In the vast living room of his house in Eldoret, he would point to a poster of himself at the finish line in Boston in 2011, with the clock frozen at 2:03:02 above his head. Smiling out from beneath his habitual porkpie hat, his puckish disposition laced with a priestly seriousness, he nodded at the photograph and said: "When I dream, I see that time."

And so Mutai set about his preparations for the London Marathon like a warrior monk. He was determined to perform well. The previous year, a week after failing to finish Boston in the warm weather, he was invited to watch the 2012 London Marathon from a pace truck. He sat, impassive in wraparound shades, and observed as his friend Wilson Kipsang picked off a strong field with two surges at halfway and 20 miles to win the race in 2:04:44. Although Mutai's expression gave little away, he said he longed to be on the road fighting for victory, instead of watching from the truck, impotent.

In the early part of 2013, Mutai's training was solid. He arrived at the Ras al-Khaimah half marathon in February in superb shape. The RAK half, as it is known, is a tune-up event for the spring marathon season and a big-money race in its own right. Mutai came in third, four seconds behind the winner, Geoffrey Kamworor, and two seconds behind Stanley Biwott. All of the top three broke 59 minutes, and their personal bests, that day. But for Mutai, the result came at a cost. Toward the end of the race, Biwott had been sitting at Mutai's back, letting the senior man press ahead, when he clipped Mutai's heel. There was a flicker of pain in Mutai's hamstring. The injury was not serious enough for him to stop, but it lingered.

That muscle strain niggled at him throughout his training for London. What's more, he thought, his competitors knew about it. As he arrived in London, Mutai was nervous and uncharacteristically withdrawn. He had no idea how his weak hamstring would stand up to the battle on Sunday morning.

— —

Before the race, the marathon cognoscenti could not pick a winner. Apart from Geoffrey Mutai, there was Kebede—perhaps the most consistent performer of all modern marathon runners—who had run a brilliant race in Chicago in October, winning in 2:04:38, and was said to have prepared well. Of the other contenders, the defending champion, Wilson Kipsang, was a favorite, even though his recent form was unknown. Having won London in 2012, he had traveled to New York in November, only to see the race canceled because of Hurricane Sandy. (He later entered and won the steamy Honolulu Marathon in a time of 2:12:31.) Biwott was an outside shot. He won the 2012 Paris Marathon in 2:05:11, a course record, and finished second in the RAK half in January in the impressive time of 58:56.

In the buildup to Sunday's event, however, the elite athletes were asked fewer questions about their prospects for the race than they might usually have expected. What reporters wanted to know, in the aftermath of Boston, was how safe the athletes felt in London, and what they thought about the atrocity. Wilson Kipsang gave a simple but touching answer. He told the press he and his fellow athletes would run "free from fear."

As the double-decker buses left from Tower Bridge to Blackheath for the start of the race, all the conversation was of a world record. History suggested that so many studs in one pack would call for a tactical race, and "tactical" generally means "slow." But there were also signs that there might be an attack on a fast time. Geoffrey Mutai's training partner Dennis Kimetto, who ran one second slower than him in Berlin, had been brought to London at Mutai's request as a pacemaker. With rabbits of that quality, it seemed possible that a plan was being formulated to run a lightning time.

According to various athletes and managers, a phony war had taken place in the official marathon hotel in the week before the race. At issue was how Sunday's marathon would be paced. Some runners wanted a 62-minute first half and others wanted a 61:45. Patrick Makau was said to be in the 62 camp, with Wilson Kipsang and Geoffrey Mutai pressing for a faster split. Not everyone was so forceful in venturing an opinion. And it was these silent athletes who would later determine the speed and shape of the race.

Whatever was eventually decided among the elite athletes, all of them must have looked out of the window that Sunday morning and known one thing: the race was going to start fast. In the minutes before the gun, the excitement among the organizers, watching journalists, coaches, and other aficionados was palpable. Dave Bedford, the impresario who had spent months and years curating the elite fields for the race, was in a gregarious mood. Talking to his friend Mark Milde, who organizes the Berlin Marathon, he looked upward at the sky and said, "If they don't want to run fast today, they'll never want to run fast." Milde then attempted a little joke.

"Okay," said Milde, "you can have the world record back, for a little while."

"We'll return it in September, I promise," said Bedford, referring to the upcoming Berlin Marathon.

Everybody laughed.

—

As the gun sounded, the lead pack was briefly surprised by an unknown competitor. A white athlete, who was not part of the elite field, sprinted the first few hundred meters ahead of the race favorites, if only to say that he had—for a time—led the London Marathon. He must have been a decent runner, otherwise he would not have started so close behind the elite, but his challenge lasted only a minute or so. As the lead men swerved to either side of a set of traffic lights, like a stream around a boulder, the phantom sprinter stopped, stooped, and caught his breath.

It was an odd moment. From the truck that drove in front of the race, where the managers and coaches of the elite runners watched the race, the reaction to this man's quest for fleeting glory was a chuckle, or a dismissive hand gesture. These men were in town for business, not japes. But the stunt was also a reminder of the otherworldly accomplishment of the elite runners. After years of witnessing the Kenyans and Ethiopians race mile after mile at a sub-5-minute pace, it was easy to become blasé about their industry and talent. The amateur's sprint briefly connected everyday runners to the elite and set their wondrous achievements in context. Somehow, the sport at large had forgotten how to communicate that sense of awe. But, for those few seconds, it returned.

The real race started fast, debilitatingly so. Early in the action, key figures from the pre-event hype were dropped from the lead group. The world record holder Patrick Makau was 40 seconds back by 10km—although, strangely, he was still nearly on his own world record pace.

At the prow of the field, it was a gorgeous sight. The proud-chested pacemakers, in black and white stripes, led out the contenders, each man arrayed in vivid colors. There was Mo Farah, in navy blue with the gold skull motif of the Nike Oregon Project rampant above his heart; the Ethiopian athletes Abshero, Lilesa, and Kebede, all decked in baby blue; Emmanuel Mutai in lurid yellow; and the burnt oranges, peaches, and reds of Wilson Kipsang, Geoffrey Mutai, and Stanley Biwott. When the group turned a corner and caught a shaft of sunlight, it was like watching a shoal of tropical fish tack against a current.

Despite the apparently serene progress of the lead group, however, breathless arguments were breaking out. The pace was not only fast, but uneven. The speed yo-yoed around over the early part of the course like the most aggressive *Fartlek* training you could imagine. Wilson Kipsang realized that what the elite men were doing in the early kilometers was suicidal—to him, at least. Geoffrey Mutai shared this view. He also maintained the (perhaps paranoid) belief that the other runners were deliberately testing his weak hamstring with their fast-slow-fast pace. In any event, these complaints were not heeded. The pacemakers were cajoled by Emmanuel Mutai to keep the coal burning.

The experience was too much for Dennis Kimetto, the star rabbit, who hurt his leg just after 6 miles and pulled out. Still, eight competitors came through the halfway mark in 61:34, well inside world record schedule. At halfway, the ninth-placed man—the unlikely Olympic champion from Uganda, Stephen Kiprotich—was adrift of the lead pack, but still running a world record pace.

The watching managers felt a sense of impending doom. It was as if the runners, through their dazzling, uneven start, were deliberately throwing themselves on a bonfire and seeing who could stand the heat the longest. This is not, traditionally, how world records are set. But it was the best way Emmanuel Mutai, a clever competitor, could see to win the race.

After the halfway mark, the leaders surged again. It was a deliberate effort to shake up the race once more, and it succeeded in that mission. Geoffrey Mutai, Wilson Kipsang, and Tsegaye Kebede dropped from the lead pack. Geoffrey knew he was gone for good. Searing pain coursed through his thigh—the injury from RAK. After soldiering on for a few miles, he eventually abandoned the race at around 20 miles and left the course in a wheelchair.

Now it was only Emmanuel, Abshero, Lelisa, and Biwott who remained in front, pushing out devastating kilometers. And, after the ludicrous surge, all of them suffered. From 25km onward, the lead changed hands several times among this quartet while the pace dropped precipitously. When the lead swapped, it was never the result of a runner making a decisive move. All four men were dying; the lead was determined by who felt least terrible. When Biwott took the front spot, he looked strong enough to finish the job and win the race, but Emmanuel eventually caught him. As Biwott's challenge ended, Emmanuel appeared destined for his second London victory.

If Emmanuel's plan had been to destroy his competitors—and a world record attempt—with punishing surges in the early and middle parts of the race, it seemed to have worked. Patrick Sang, his coach, stood up in the truck and pumped his fist as his athlete ran alone down London's Embankment. But then his athlete, like the rest, felt concrete in his legs. Behind him, the tiny Ethiopian Kebede was quietly covering the ground at a steadier pace. To Kebede's great surprise, he began overtaking athletes he thought had forged an insuperable lead. Emmanuel came into his sights in the final mile. Kebede caught him, overtook him, and won the marathon in 2:06:04, 26 seconds ahead of the Kenyan.

After the race, some of the other runners were angry at Emmanuel Mutai. Great athletes had either been knocked out cold or had limped home in times they would be embarrassed to run in training. The world record holder Patrick Makau, for instance, finished in 2:14 and change. Meanwhile, as Kipsang splashed cold water on his head after a fifth-place finish, he said, "Emmanuel was pushing, pushing! Too much! If we could run 62 for the first half, and go as a group to 30km, we could run two-oh-three or two-oh-four today." Or, as Geoffrey Mutai had it: "He kills everybody, and then he kills himself."

But that was the reality of racing. Emmanuel Mutai had no commercial interest in letting a pack of eight or nine of the finest distance runners on the planet run an even pace, so that they reached the final stages of the marathon in great shape. He wanted to boss the race. The London Marathon, he understood, was not a time trial but a competition. Kebede, the Ethiopian who finally bested Emmanuel, and a pure racer himself, recognized the bravery of the attempt. In the tent by the finishing line, he looked at his tormentor with a smile and said, "Mutai, you killed me!"

The next day, the other Mutai, Geoffrey, went for a slow jog in the dull early morning, just to move his weary limbs. He then went back to bed for a long time. Once he had woken at around lunchtime, the pain not only of his injury, but of a missed opportunity, began to register. He tried to analyze the marathon as he saw it. He said that the pace, spurred by Emmanuel and Biwott, was "faster, slower" and it was hard to resist such a pace when one was feeling tight. His failure had been a grave disappointment, but he was determined to rebuild himself once more. In his head, he still saw his landmark time, 2:03:02, and longed to best it.

"You will see," he said. "I will perform again."

———

Five months later, Geoffrey Mutai was at home in Eldoret, waiting to watch his friend Kipsang run the Berlin Marathon on television. He and Kipsang were friends and colleagues, as well as rivals. Both men were managed by Gerard Van de Veen. Occasionally, Kipsang would travel the two hours from Iten to Kapng'tuny for some serious training. After London, Van de Veen had asked them both which fall marathon they would prefer to run.

The question was loaded. It made little sense for Van de Veen to have his two best runners compete against one another. Financially, it was preferable for the two of them to race, and win, in different marathons. So, if Kipsang ran Berlin, there was no chance of Mutai joining him. And Kipsang had been eyeing the Berlin Marathon for a while, ever since he missed the world record by four seconds in Frankfurt in 2011.

Mutai, meanwhile, loved New York, even though there was no chance of running a world record there. It had been the site of his greatest performance, the 2:05:06 in 2011, and because of the cancellation of the New York City Marathon in 2012 due to Hurricane Sandy, he was still the reigning champion. Van de Veen came up with an equitable solution. Kipsang would go to Germany in September to attempt the world record, Mutai to the United States in November to defend his title. (Kimetto, the other star in Van de Veen's stable, was scheduled to race in Chicago, meaning it was possible for all three fall Majors to be won by Van de Veen's athletes.)

Still, Mutai grew uneasy at the thought of watching anyone—even his friend—achieve something magical in Berlin. On the morning of the race, he was sitting on his favorite sofa, with his satellite TV tuned to the right channel, his family by his side, and every comfort at hand. But it seemed wrong, somehow, to watch the marathon in that setting. So he drove into town to meet up with other athletes at La Clique, a popular, somewhat grubby bar on the main drag. He was met there by Kimetto, his taciturn training mate, as well as Stephen Kiprotich, the Ugandan Olympic and world champion, and Ezekiel Kemboi, the Mohawked Olympic gold medalist in the steeplechase.

In the bar, the athletes were excited at the prospect of a world record. Wilson Kipsang would compete with two outstanding athletes from Jos Hermens's Global group: Eliud Kipchoge, a track star running his second marathon, and Geoffrey Kamworor, the young bull of whom so much was expected. Mutai watched the flickering images from Berlin and felt as he often did while watching races on television: as if his heart might burst.

With a minute to go, Kipsang stood at the startline in an orange-red vest and blue shorts. He rocked his head from side to side, to loosen his neck muscles. Mutai knew that feeling: the attempt to focus, to relax, to somehow connect the body to the moment. He watched as Kipsang smiled broadly—that handsome toothy smile—and then closed his eyes for a moment. That retrenchment, too, was familiar to Mutai: the collection of one's thoughts, the banishment of extraneous noise.

Seconds to go. The two Nike athletes, Geoffrey Kamworor and Eliud Kipchoge, both wearing baby blue, stood stock-still, and then tucked into a shallow crouch. Haile Gebrselassie, booked as the celebrity starter, had his hand on the starter's gun, and the man with a microphone counted down the final seconds. *Five, four, three, two . . .*

Kipsang made a false start. He was gone with at least a second left on the countdown, but it's impossible to restart a marathon. Once Kipsang moved, nobody was inclined to allow him any extra advantage. The lead pack shot off and quickly assembled itself, with all the major players present, and a handful of Kenyan and Ethiopian athletes for whom the pace would eventually, inevitably, prove too arduous.

They began the race thrillingly fast: 14:33 for 5km, 29:16 for 10km. They hit 15km at 43:45, 35 seconds inside world record pace. Kipsang, Kamworor, and Kipchoge were all apparently comfortable. Their faces looked relaxed, as if they were simply in the early stages of a Saturday long run, conserving energy for hills to come. The lead group cruised through halfway in 61:32, just about right for a time of 2 hours, 3 minutes, dead. Had they taken the first half too fast? In London, a 61:34 opening split, followed by a surge, stunned the record attempt in its tracks. In Berlin, however, the pacing was even, and there seemed to be no appetite for a surge. It was possible that history was in the making.

But just as that thought entered the minds of spectators in the Eldoret bar, the record attempt appeared to stall. In the third quarter of the race, the three main contenders relaxed the pace, apparently wary of each other. They were now racing alone, and each man waited for the other to make a move. By 27km, the pace had slowed enough that the lead group was seven seconds outside the world record—a significant swing from the position at halfway. Watching on the television, Mutai thought, *Come on! You are losing, you are losing!*

By 30km, Wilson Kipsang had idled long enough. Accelerating out of a drinks station, he tried to shatter the group. Geoffrey Kamworor followed the move stride for stride. Kipchoge, a more experienced athlete, accelerated more gently and gradually made up the ground. At 32km, Wilson Kipsang, now in attack mode, teeth beginning to show, ran past a spectator holding a sign that said, "Hurry! Das Bier Wird Warm!"—"Hurry! The Beer's Getting Warm!"

Kipsang needed no encouragement. Kipchoge and Kamworor were still on his tail. He maintained his killer pace and eventually the group broke. At 33km, Kamworor began to rock and roll with his powerful shoulders, a sign that he was about to fall away. Kipchoge, his hangdog face now taut with concentration, appeared to be working hard to maintain a connection with Wilson. All the while, the tall, leggy leader kept his hands low and his shoulders down and attempted to maintain his rhythm.

Mutai understood the anguish, and the effort, intimately. He was one of only a handful of people who could ever know what it was like to run so fast, so late in the marathon: banishing doubt, pinning one's thoughts solely to the finish line, *fighting inside*. Now, in his mind, he ran every stride with Kipsang.

By 35km there were 15 meters between the first two men, and the pace was slightly underneath world record schedule. Kipchoge looked as if he might still mount a challenge, but Kipsang kept pushing, and the gap increased, meter by meter. At 40km, Wilson looked at the clock on the pace car. It read: 1:57:12. He made a quick calculation. In Frankfurt, in 2011, he had passed 40km in 1:57:20, but missed the world record by four seconds.

Kipsang was determined to be satisfied this time. With the record within reach, he picked up his knees and drummed his feet against the tarmac. With 400 meters to go, he passed underneath the four-horsed chariot at the Brandenburg Gate alone, and drove toward the line, hands still low, legs hammering.

As Mutai watched in La Clique, he felt as he did a decade earlier, when nobody knew him as an athlete, and he used to watch track meets on television. He broke out in sweats. Mutai wanted his colleague to succeed, but he also reflected on his own disappointments from the previous year. His effort in Berlin in 2012 had been plagued by technical difficulties, an injury, and— possibly—a lack of premium shape. Now his friend was going to break a world record, if not Mutai's own "world best" time of 2:03:02 from Boston. He felt a curious mixture of pride, joy, and wistfulness.

Kipsang crested the line in 2 hours, 3 minutes, and 23 seconds—a new world record by 15 seconds. Just before he did so, a plump middle-aged man advertising a prostitution service across a lurid yellow vest jumped out from behind a barrier and ran the final meters with Kipsang. This interloper raised his hands a second before Kipsang, ruining a hundred front-page photographs, and was soon wrestled to the ground by security guards. But Kipsang hardly seemed to notice him. Having stumbled a little, the new world-record holder regathered himself and set off with a Kenyan flag draped around his shoulders to celebrate with the crowd.

The atmosphere in La Clique was jubilant. Another world record had fallen to one of their own. Mutai stayed awhile, talking with his friends, before driving home. In the hours, days, and weeks after Kipsang's run, this one thought would not leave him: "It was so easy, how he did it."

Chapter Ten

Broken Stones

November 2013: Before, and Ever After

O N THE afternoon of November 2, 2013, more than six months after his disappointment in London, and five weeks after Kipsang's world record in Berlin, Geoffrey Mutai peered out the window of his hotel room on the thirty-second floor of the Hilton hotel in midtown Manhattan. He had an uninterrupted view north to Central Park. From this eyrie, the park's thinning canopy of dull yellow and brown leaves looked too perfect—like an architect's model of some future city. In less than a day's time, it would seem real enough to Mutai. The New York City Marathon finished in the park. It would be the site of either his triumph or his failure.

That afternoon, with nothing to do but hang around the hotel and wait until race day, Mutai had other things on his mind. Crazy things had already happened in the fall marathon season. Not only had Kipsang sliced fifteen seconds out of Makau's record, but, two weeks later at the Chicago Marathon, Mutai's training partner Dennis "Mwafrica" Kimetto had won in 2:03:45 after a brutal duel with Emmanuel Mutai, who finished seven seconds behind, in 2:03:52. Two-oh-three marathons were becoming commonplace.

Mutai was now in New York with no such prospect. He had arrived in the city earlier in the week in a bullish mood, having run a 59-minute half marathon in Italy as a tune-up. At a press conference, he predicted he would break his own course record from two years earlier and run New York's first two-oh-four marathon on the way to defending his title.

A low pressure system advancing toward the city seemed destined to spoil that plan. A strong, freezing wind was forecast to blow from the north, meaning the runners would be fighting the breeze for 20 miles until they turned south in the Bronx. New York is always a slow course, with its hills and bridges and its lack of pacemakers, but the foul weather would make it a slog. The winning athlete would have to make canny decisions and tough it out. Mutai could run that kind of race, but it was not what thrilled him.

In his hotel room, he walked gingerly in his stocking feet to the bed and sat down. There was boxing on the television, muted. After everything that had happened in his racing life since his glorious 2011, Mutai wanted the win in New York more than anything. Kipsang's achievement had redoubled his ambition. He told himself with pride that nobody, not even the new world record holder, had run faster than his 2:03:02 at Boston. He still wished to claim the crown he believed was his by right.

His likely schedule of future marathons, however, gave him few opportunities to do so. He was in his early thirties, approaching the end of the peak of his career. Tomorrow would be his thirteenth professional marathon. Very few people improved after ten marathons, and most didn't improve after six. Makau and Tergat broke the world record in their sixth marathons. Kipsang and Haile, both relatively slow starters, broke the record in their seventh. (And Haile broke it again in his ninth.)

Perversely, Mutai's success impinged on his ambitions. While there were a handful of second-tier courses that were tailor-made for fast times—Eindhoven, Dubai, Rotterdam, and so on—he would run none of them in the near future. Mutai's status as a marathoner had padlocked him to the Majors. Practically, that meant that he would run New York tomorrow, where there was no chance of a world record, and London in the spring, where the chances were vanishingly small. And who knew where he would be next fall? It would depend on how he fared in New York and London. Whatever happened, it was possible his chance to become the world's first two-oh-two guy had come and gone in Berlin the previous year.

Mutai would not accept it. He stood up from the bed, walked to the window, and looked up Sixth Avenue toward the park again. As he spoke on these matters, his jocular demeanor thinned. Briefly lost in thought, he appeared as he does when he attempts to press in a race: his head dipped, his nostrils flared, and his lips curled into the suggestion of a grimace. Returning to sit at the end of his double bed, in a $600-a-night room in the heart of the world's most famous metropolis, thousands of miles from his unshod past, he refused to acknowledge that his moment was gone.

"I still have time," he said. There was no doubt in his voice. "I still have time."

——

When Tiger Woods was eighteen years old, having been voted "Most Likely to Succeed" by his high school colleagues, he enrolled at Stanford University on a golf scholarship. He won his first collegiate championship within weeks. When Roger Federer was eighteen years old, he was making his way on the ATP tour as a professional tennis player. In his first tour final, in Marseilles, he wept openly when he lost to an older opponent. When Lionel Messi was eighteen years old, he was already a member of Barcelona's first team squad. He received a standing ovation from fans in the 96,000-seat Camp Nou stadium when he was substituted near the end of his first Champions League match, against Udinese.

When Geoffrey Mutai was eighteen, he broke rocks. In Kenya, they use small stones called *kokoto* to fortify cement for building roads and houses. For the stones to be useful, they need to be roughly marble-sized and more or less regular in shape. You can go about making *kokoto* two ways: with industrial equipment, or using strong-backed young men with hammers. In Rongai, where Mutai spent much of his childhood, they did it the old-fashioned way.

At that moment in Mutai's life, his prospects were uninviting. The idea that he might one day become famous, or rich, would have been laughable. The eldest sibling in a poor family, he was struggling to graduate from primary school, even in his late teens. He sometimes drank too much. His abusive father, meanwhile, seemed to sense a challenge to his authority in every decision his son took. He had received beatings of every kind. But Mutai was also ambitious and, despite struggling to see out of his current predicament, he wanted to finish school, however old he was for his grade. Rock-breaking paid for uniforms and examination fees, which his parents could not afford.

Mutai remembers that those days in the quarry were killing. First, you had to break a big rock with a sledgehammer. Then you'd use a smaller hammer, a *nyundo*, to smash those chunks into the gravel-like *kokoto*. You were paid according to volume. One full, coffin-sized plastic container paid ten shillings—about a quarter of a dollar. Even if he worked at his hardest, the most containers he could hope to fill in a day was six. That was his limit: a dollar fifty. At the end of the day, with his back aching and blisters on his hands, he would help the other boys load the heavy boxes into the tractor before walking home.

Long before Mutai became a runner, he knew what it meant to work and was adept at the management of pain. He had never forgotten what it felt like to suffer. He understood that true pain is not the kind felt by athletes, which is merely physiological, but the pain that comes with the suppression of your life chances. He knew that in order to become a runner he had needed first to become a man. *Nobody was born with anything*, he had told himself. *Get up. Work.*

As an athlete, Mutai approached his training in the same manner in which he had labored in the quarry as a teenager: Smash as many rocks as you can, then return the next day and do the same. Week after week, month after month, break the stones and fill the boxes. The Spirit, as he understood it—that electrifying feeling of pure athletic expression, which he had experienced only a handful of times—was summoned by such quotidian drudgery.

By the time of the 2013 New York City Marathon he had been

in near-constant training for more than a decade. The results of his labor had been extraordinary. He had won some of the world's most prestigious races and become the fastest marathoner in the history of the sport. But, despite these achievements, he continued to grope in the dark for something he did not possess.

Being a great marathoner, he now realized, was not simply a question of breaking stones. His sport prized special moments. There were days in marathon running that weighed more than the others—races that could change everything. And how those days appeared in your life seemed as connected to luck—or God, perhaps—as your own best efforts. Industry was rewarded sometimes, but not always. You ran 2:03:02 in Boston and everybody talked about the wind. Then, in the best shape of your career, you ran New York—an impossible course on which to break the world record. When you had your chance in Berlin the following year to claim what you believed was yours by right, the clocks froze and your hamstring pinched.

By his own exacting standards, Mutai had still not proved himself.

——

Sometimes, at night in his hilltop training camp, Mutai thought about a new kind of race. He longed to know the ultimate performance within his body. He wanted to understand whether he was truly capable of the speed he believed he possessed. And so he imagined an event whose only purpose was to see what was possible—a moonshot whose sole purpose was *time*.

In Mutai's head, the New Race went like this: You got a few strong guys together and then you built them a course somewhere flat and out of the wind. Teams of pacemakers would come in and out of the race, circuit by circuit, right until the end, so that the runners had company and protection all the way. And everybody got paid if one of them broke a record. "Organize it like that," he said, on one such night, "and I will sacrifice myself to that level. Even to run sub-two hours is possible. People can run crazy times."

Mutai is not the only person to have thought in this way. Mike Joyner, of the Mayo Clinic, believes that once the world record reaches 2:02 and change, record breaking will become the preserve of specialist time trials like the one Mutai outlined. In 2011, he suggested the idea to Jos Hermens, the manager of—among others—Haile Gebrselassie.

Hermens was fascinated. He has always been interested in unconventional events, and new ways of thinking about the sport. As an athlete, he twice broke a seldom-contested world record for the one-hour run, an event that tests the total distance an athlete can run in an hour on the track. Everybody had forgotten about the one-hour record until Hermens came along and broke it in 1976 and 1977. But he was a student of the sport. Paavo Nurmi, Emil Zátopek, and Ron Clarke, who were all heroes to Hermens, had all broken the record. He wanted to join that list. Years later, as Haile's manager, he convinced the Ethiopian to give it a shot. Haile shattered the one-hour best: one of twenty-seven world records he set in his career.

The moonshot marathon is a development of the one-hour-run idea—a two-hour run, if you like—and it has played on Hermens's mind awhile. "I've got a lot of ideas," he said. "You've got to be in the woods, so there's a lot of oxygen. Think about the shoes, the asphalt. Maybe there's some new material we haven't thought about yet. The climate has to be right. It has to be a loop.

The trouble is, it would cost a lot. But if the world record gets to 2.01, and someone puts in ten million . . ."

Hermens is right. Designing the mechanics and economics of such a world record attempt would be complex. You'd need a ton of money because you'd need four or five of the best runners in the world as well as a string of excellent rabbits. By committing to the world record time trial, they would be missing a marathon—and potentially a few hundred thousand dollars in appearance fees, as well as a shot at the World Marathon Majors jackpot—so whatever you offered them would need to be substantial. In order to promote a team effort, you would pay all your star athletes the same bonus if one of them broke 2:03, more if one broke 2:02:30, and so on. You might also pay them for hitting particular splits during the attempt. The pacers would also be recompensed, at a lower level, for their part in making history.

This structure might overcome many of the factors that inhibit fast times in city marathons. Instead of setting a single date, and then running on that day whatever the weather, you could aim for a window of a few days and then choose the perfect day of that period: windless and chilly. Elite athletes create much more body heat than amateur runners, and the ideal temperature for the world's best to run a fast marathon, according to recent research conducted in France, is 38.9 degrees Fahrenheit. Very few Majors ever take place in such frigid conditions.

You might also run your time trial in the evening. City marathons are largely run in the morning for the simple logistical reason that they're easier to arrange then. But it's possible elite athletes might run faster in the evening. Not only would the day be cooling down as the athletes are heating up, but they might naturally run better at dusk because of their circadian rhythms. Several studies have shown that athletes perform marginally better in the early evening. (Plus, as anyone who has watched footage of Abebe Bikila's triumph through the uplit Rome streets in 1960 will know, it is profoundly dramatic to watch a marathon as day turns to night.)

You might also want to mess with the athletes' heads a little. In Kevin Thompson's study, cyclists on a bike machine pushed beyond their perceived limits while racing an avatar that they believed represented their personal best, but was in fact a little faster. You might squeeze an extra second per kilometer out of runners that way, although you might have to revert to the "correct" time nearer the end if the athletes looked close to breaking a significant landmark. People trying to break records push themselves harder if they believe they can really do it. You don't want to screw with them *too* much.

The chief obstacle is money. It's also not easy to see how the major marathon circuit would agree to being interrupted by the moonshot marathon. On the other hand, it's not difficult to imagine who might gain from such an event. The Adidas shoe designers said that as part of their more general "sub-two" conversation, they had discussed a time trial remarkably similar to the one Mutai outlined. And consider if Adidas *did* decide to hold such a race. Some of the fastest marathoners in the world are signed to their stable. Imagine if Geoffrey and Emmanuel Mutai, Wilson Kipsang, and Dennis Kimetto were all recruited to the time trial—and if they were all committed to a team effort?

To a promoter with imagination, the event could be a singular commercial opportunity. One of the elements that has helped to save interest in professional boxing is the prefight documentary show. Before an anticipated bout, HBO runs a series called *24/7* that spends time in the boxers' camps and films their physical and mental preparations in a verité style. Ever since the series began with Oscar De La Hoya versus Floyd Mayweather Jr. in 2007, fans have eaten it up. Similarly, anticipation for the "Two Hour Project"—or whatever you wanted to call it—could be generated with footage from training and tune-up races, visits from motivational speakers, commentary from sports scientists, and so on.

Naturally, none of this is likely to happen soon. The moon-shot idea is antithetical to the conservative ethos and spirit of the marathon. It's not in the DNA of distance running, or its most able proponents, to make a big show. (As David Hannah, the former director of the Houston Marathon, once wryly observed, "A long time ago, running made an unconscious decision to be a closely held secret.") Done badly, the moonshot could be a disaster. You'd need to monitor the legitimacy of any such event by drug testing the athletes regularly. Done right, however, it could transform interest in the marathon.

In 1908, during marathon mania, Dorando Pietri and Johnny Hayes sold out Madison Square Garden for a two-man marathon footrace of 262 laps each. Objectively, what they were doing—running, not very fast, around the Garden—was deathly boring. But the event was charged with meaning. People wanted to see Pietri and Hayes race again because of the drama of their earlier encounter in London. Now imagine watching the world's greatest athletes shoot for the two-hour marathon. To purists, the moonshot, which would break about a dozen IAAF rules, would be a perversion of the sport. To others, it would be the sport's ultimate distillation.

We are hardwired to discover new ways to test ourselves. The urge resides somewhere in our traveler genes. Whatever science or common sense one uses to rebut the possibility of a two-hour marathon, we still cannot resist its lure. Everest was unclimbable until somebody climbed it. The four-minute mile was impossible until it wasn't. However evanescent the prospect, the two-hour marathon will not leave us alone.

—

Mutai looked out of the window on the frigid, breezy morning of November 3 and knew there was no chance of a fast time. Whatever thoughts he had entertained about new races, and old ones—of records and his place in athletic history—he would need to park them. The win would need to be enough. This thought, in fact, was liberating for Mutai. As he completed his final warm-up shuttle runs on the Verrazano-Narrows Bridge in his electric-orange and blue Adidas uniform, he looked sleek and bright-eyed.

Into the stiff wind, the race started slow. A large pack, including Tsegaye Kebede, Stephen Kiprotich, and Stanley Biwott, made it to halfway in a little over 1 hour and 5 minutes: on track for a 2:10 finish. During that first half, Mutai spent much of his time idling at the back of the group, out of the breeze. He was the only man in the lead pack not wearing some kind of arm or hand protection against the bitter wind, and it appeared he was trying to stay warm.

At halfway, the pace was sluggish, and Mutai attempted to scatter the field with a trademark burst of pace. But, for once in his professional life, the speed did not come. He pressed on the mental accelerator, but there was no juice in his legs. "The body

did not respond," he remembered later, amused, like a man re-
calling his travails with a faulty truck.

Perhaps he was simply too cold, he thought. He tried to increase his cadence steadily, to generate pace by degrees. This
seemed to work. He warmed up. But at mile 17, cruising north
on First Avenue, there was still a pack of nine men in the lead
group. Too many. Mutai prepared himself for another assault,
praying his body would react this time to his instructions. At
mile 20, in the Bronx, the group began to turn west, and then
south. For the first time in the race, the wind was with them.
Mutai picked his moment and began his attack. This time, his
body reacted with gusto. The field all but shattered.

Only one man withstood the attack: Stanley Biwott. Mutai
knew Biwott was a threat. He had scorched a Paris Marathon
win in 2012 with a course record of 2:05:12, and had been leading the crazy London race earlier in the year until the final miles.
At the RAK half marathon, Biwott had been the man who kicked
Mutai's leg from behind, causing the hamstring strain that became the injury that forced him out of London in a wheelchair.
He was damned if Biwott was going to do it again. As the two
men ran alone down Fifth Avenue, with clear air between them
and the challengers, Mutai told Biwott to come alongside him
rather than loiter behind. Biwott assented. They strode through
Harlem side by side.

At the final drinks station, just before 22 miles, Biwott missed
his bottle of water. It was, both men knew, the last station before
the end, so Mutai offered his bottle to Biwott: a gracious gesture,
but not an uncommon one in the pro marathon. It was the second time Mutai had talked to Biwott within the space of a half

mile—and was perhaps a subliminal reminder from the senior man to his junior of which one of them had won three major marathons and which of them had won none.

Four miles to go. Whatever mind games he was playing, Mutai knew he'd have to attack again if he wanted to win the race. And he needed to win the race. He steeled himself for another burst. At 107th Street and Fifth, it came. Mutai's head dipped—the look that said *now, business*—his legs whirred, the edges of his shorts rippled. The gap between him and Biwott opened like a torn shirt. In fact, as soon as the burst came, the younger athlete immediately turned his head to see who was behind him. Now Mutai was leading by an unassailable margin, heart racing, arms low and pumping. The Spirit coursed through him.

"I didn't notice anyone," he would say afterward, and looking at him, you could believe it. There was no thought of world records, course records, goals, demons, splits. He did not think of the next race or the runners who were behind him. It was just him, alone, on Fifth Avenue. He had become the workings of his own body.

It was in these moments that Mutai was happiest, most fully himself. He was always less interested in the products of running—the cars, the houses, the wealth and its associated burdens—than in the act itself. There was joy in running fast, and freedom in it too. The process connected him not only to his own past but to the sport's. How many other champions—Pietri, Bikila, Zátopek, Clayton—had felt this coursing Spirit, late in great races? Mutai was no historian, and he didn't know the names of every giant who had come before him, but he intimately understood their experience. Right now, he was an athlete and an athlete only. Right now, he felt the supreme comfort of a talent redeemed, the expression of a gift he believed to have come from God. He had suffered real pain—lasting pain—to be here. He had broken rocks, walked through a burning village. And now he was flying through the Manhattan streets, approaching glory.

Mutai savored these numinous minutes. He would need the memory of them when, six months later, while leading the 2014 London Marathon, he felt a stomach cramp knot and stifle his insides and crawled to a sixth-place finish. He would need them as he watched his friend Kipsang soak up the attention that attended his win in London; as he sat broken in the tarpaulin athletes' tent at the finish line in the shadow of Buckingham Palace alongside his wife and youngest daughter. Mutai would need to summon strength from somewhere, and the joy he felt on Fifth Avenue would always sustain him.

Mutai crested the tape in Central Park to cheers and gloved applause from the freezing spectators. He raised his arms in triumph. It was his fourth Major: the same number reached by his hero, Haile Gebrselassie. To most spectators, the numbers on the clock above Mutai's head as he finished, 2:08:24, were irrelevant. Everyone knew the conditions had been atrocious. But Mutai, gnawed as he was by the Boston demon and driven by forces even he only dimly understood, could never be fully satisfied with a two-oh-eight. Victory, however, was a powerful physic. A champion once more, he wrapped himself in his nation's flag, flashed his gleaming teeth, and set off to celebrate with the crowd.

That night, once his duties with the press were fulfilled, Mutai ate dinner with his manager, drank a little wine, and shared tales from the old days—good stories, happy stories. He was cheerful. The New York finish line, he knew, was not the end. He would feel the Spirit again. He remained the fastest marathoner in history, and could go faster still.

Yes, he thought, *I still have time.*

Postscript

AT THE 2014 Berlin Marathon, Geoffrey Mutai's training mate Dennis Kimetto set a new world record of 2:02:57. The time not only beat Wilson Kipsang's previous world record of 2:03:23, which was set in Berlin the previous year, but Mutai's "world best" of 2:03:02, set at the 2011 Boston Marathon.

Five weeks later, in freezing windy conditions, Geoffrey Mutai placed sixth in 2:13:44 at the New York City Marathon.

On December 17, 2014, in Newcastle, England, a group led by Yannis Pitsiladis, PhD, launched the Sub2hr Project to "identify and nurture" a runner who could break two hours within the next five years.

Acknowledgments

I SIGNED a contract to write this book in December 2011. I'm writing these acknowledgments in December 2014. Plenty's happened in those three years: I've moved houses twice; I've witnessed a lynching; I've eaten dinner with Roger Federer. My son Rory—who was not conceived when I began working on the book—has become a cheeky, delightful toddler who says things like "What are you *talking* about, Daddy?" And, somehow, I've also completed *Two Hours*.

I would not have made it without the help and love of a large number of people. Thank you to my family, in particular my beautiful and patient wife, Chloë. It is indisputable that I could not have written this book without you. Rory, life has been so much more fun since you've been around. Thank you, gorgeous boy. Mum, Peter, Dave, Ben, Claire, Lotte, Jamie, Gabriel, Hattie, and the rest of Team Caesar—I love you all. Judith, RTJ, Theo, and Ponny: thanks for the sausages, the reading chair, and your many other kindnesses.

At Curtis Brown, my profound gratitude to Karolina Sutton—doyenne of agents, agent of doyens—who asked in 2008 whether I had a book in me. She has waited longer than most to discover the answer. Also, thank you to Sloan Harris at ICM, who told me when we first met to "make a big bet" on myself. I followed his advice. Let's see how it works out.

Jofie Ferrari-Adler, my editor at Simon & Schuster, changed my life. Because of his early and enthusiastic support for this book, he allowed me the freedom to quit my newspaper contract and write big stories. I can't thank him enough for his encouragement, and for the tough love he metes out with the blue pen. My warmest thanks also to Joel Rickett in London, another early believer in this book, who has been a font of optimism.

Many friends have offered advice to me throughout the writing of *Two Hours*. Tom Williams and Lauren Collins—both superb writers—have read every draft. I am so grateful for their generosity and kindly bedside manner. Michael Joyner and Toni Reavis have not only contributed to my understanding of the physiology and history of the sport of marathon running throughout my research, but have also read the book to check it for factual accuracy. Thank you both for everything.

Many others have supported and encouraged me throughout my development as a writer, from my unpromising beginnings as the author of god-awful teenage poetry to now. Among them are: Chris Craig, Kevin Shillington, Anne and Jonty Driver, Peter Shilston, Mike Fox, Ken Millard, Adam Leigh, Ruth Metzstein, Simon Kelner, Jo Ellison, Robin Morgan, David James Smith, Sarah Baxter, Dylan Jones, Jonathan Heaf, Alex Bilmes, Andrew Holgate, Kate Bucknell, Hugo Lindgren, Brendan Koerner, Philip Gourevitch, and Daniel Zalewski.

Colum McCann has taken me in, in every sense, and I'm so grateful for his advice, whiskey, and spare room. Robin and Penny Dyer treated me like family for five years and will always be family to me. Carne and Karmen Ross have given me a bed, great company, and world-class bagels in New York. The Hotel Roscoe was another great Manhattan establishment: thank you Clemency and James for your frequent generosity. In London, I have been grateful for the distractions offered by my officemates, particularly the old lags: Riz, Nick, Debora, and Simon. Also, my love to all the wizards of NW10 and beyond.

At the Berlin Marathon, Mark Milde got me as close to the action as was humanly possible. David Bedford at the London Marathon also steamrolled protocol to give me the access I needed. Thank you both so much. Thank you too to the athlete managers who let me pester their stars: Gerard Van de Veen, Valentijn Trouw, Jos Hermens, and Federico Rosa.

In Kenya, I am grateful to the owners and staff of the Kerio View hotel in Iten, who laughably let me pay the "athlete rate" during my many visits. In Nairobi, Wil, Flora, Zara, and Miles showed me wonderful hospitality. In Eldoret, many thanks to Claudio Berardelli, who was kind enough to offer me his spare room any time I needed it. I also ate a lot of his excellent *penne al'arrabiata*. Thank you too to all the athletes who gave me so much of their time and their tea while I reported *Two Hours*. In particular, I should thank Wilson Kipsang and Geoffrey Kamworor, with whom I spent a lot of time, but whose stories are not prominent in the book. Also, thanks Wilson for fixing my car and teaching me how to repair a faulty starter motor.

Finally, my eternal thanks to Geoffrey Mutai. This is in large part your story, and it could not have been written had you not been so open and generous. You have taught me many things, and not only about running. I feel honored that I am known to you as *Muzungu Mkubwa*: the Big White Guy.

Lea-by-Backford, England, December 2014

Notes

Two Hours is the product of three years of reporting and hundreds of interviews. In particular, the sections where Geoffrey Mutai features most prominently are guided by the many interviews I conducted with him, and by the time I spent with him at his training camp, at home, and at races in Europe and America. It should be noted that Mutai is an autodidact. He barely finished primary school and speaks English as a third language. As a result, his English is idiosyncratic. Sometimes, he makes simple errors, like confusing "he" for "she." In this book, some of those mistakes have been corrected for the sake of clarity, but some remain to give a truer impression of his speech.

It should be clear from the text where most of the information in the book comes from, but where it is not, I hope these notes will provide that sourcing and bibliographical material. These notes also contain some extra detail, which might explain certain aspects of the story more fully.

Chapter One   Tear Down This Wall

3 *Mutai is a Kenyan:* The Kipsigis are a subtribe of the Kalenjin, who are one of the forty-two tribes of Kenya.

4 *The French cyclist Jean Bobet:* Jean Bobet, *Tomorrow, We Ride* (Norwich, England: Mousehold Press, 2008).

5 *Within a few hundred:* The black-and-white striped vests are the colors of the Shaftesbury Barnet Harriers, a small running club in North Lon-

don. The London Marathon race organizer, David Bedford—a Shaftesbury Barnet Harrier man himself—decided to use them to distinguish
pacemakers from ordinary competitors in the mid-2000s. The trend has
caught on.

5 *Dennis Kimetto had been "discovered"*: There was a widely circulated
story in the Kenyan and international press that Kimetto joined Mutai's
group in 2010, having never trained a day in his life. The story went
that before he met Mutai, he was a "simple farmhand" who thought he
might have some talent for running, but had never taken training seriously. Two years later, he was breaking world records and challenging
for major marathon titles. Kimetto, a shy man with almost no English,
was in no position to rebut this narrative. But the truth was that Kimetto
had been an athlete for a long time, training either on his own or in
less recognized groups, and had won competitive races in Kenya. While
struggling with injuries, he worked on farms to earn a livelihood. He
joined Mutai's camp in around 2008, but his preparation for elite performance began years earlier. He competed at the World Junior Cross
Country Championships in 2011, where he placed fifth. As Mutai said,
"Nobody wins a race in Kenya without training. So tell me how Dennis
won those races before?"

5 *Of the contenders in Berlin*: Geoffrey Kipsang Kamworor is of no relation
to Wilson Kipsang Kiprotich. Many people in the Rift Valley Province,
where most of the world's best marathoners live, have similar names.
Some choose to go by their first and second names when racing (like
Wilson Kipsang) and some by their first and third (like Geoffrey Mutai).
In order to distinguish between them, I identify each runner by his racing name unless the context is obvious.

6 *Geoffrey Mutai is a paragon*: The slow-motion video of Geoffrey Mutai
at the New York City Marathon is available here: http://www.youtube
.com/watch?v=B4Uu3Tg71b4.

8 *"It was something incredible"*: Bill Rodgers's 2:09:55 at the 1975 Boston
Marathon was an American record.

8 *When the IAAF stipulated*: The full IAAF rules are available at http://
www.aimsworldrunning.org/IAAF_rule_260.28.htm.

9 *At 30km, he read*: Mutai was right not to trust his eyes when he looked
at the split at 30km. He recalls seeing a split of 1 hour, 26 minutes, and

several seconds. The official split was 1:28:24, which projected a finishing time of 2:04:19. In fact, the really fast running came in the next stages of the race, when Mutai scorched two absurd 5km splits of 14:12 and 14:13.

16 *Within his body, there:* Mutai has never worn a heart rate monitor in a race, but the estimation about his heart rate during the Berlin Marathon is predicated on research that says elite marathoners can sustain more than 80 percent of maximum heart rate for long periods.

16 *In his cells:* The body of a marathoner is burning so much fuel that it becomes a furnace on the move. Professionals sweat like a fat man in a sauna. During his 2007 world record run in Berlin in 2007, Haile Gebrselassie lost 10 percent of his body weight during the 2 hours, 4 minutes, and 29 seconds he was on the course. Heat, then, is one of the significant limiting factors in marathon times. For that reason, scientists are now looking into the effect of "ice slushy" drinks to cool athletes as they run. The results of such trials—at the University of Sydney and the University of Singapore—are encouraging, but it's unlikely Kenyan runners will be drinking ice slushies any time soon. They abhor cold drinks, believing it gives them stomach problems. Even in hot weather, they prefer their sodas to be served at room temperature.

Chapter Two **The Dreamers Among Us**

21 *In the last mile:* Joyner's personal bests: 14:38 for 5,000m, 30:48 for 10,000m, 2:25:44 for the marathon. Not bad for a six-foot-five guy.

22 *He'd been working on papers:* An updated version of Joyner's 1991 study was published in 2010 by the *Journal for Applied Physiology:* http://jap .physiology.org/content/early/2010/08/05/japplphysiol.00563.2010.

23 *In 2003, for instance:* Under new IAAF rules about the shape and size of the course—regulations that would exclude Geoffrey Mutai's Boston performance eight years later—Tergat's 2:04:55 was the first time to be recognized by the authorities as an official world record.

25 *Tim Noakes, one of the world's:* Tim Noakes, *Lore of Running* (Champaign, IL: Leisure Press, 1991).

25 *In 2011, at around:* Thompson et al., "Effects of Deception on Exercise Performance: Implications for Determinants of Fatigue in Humans," School of Life Sciences, University of Northumbria, 2011, http://www.re

searchgate.net/publication/51613976_Effects_of_deception_on_exercise
_performance_implications_for_determinants_of_fatigue_in_humans.

27 *The Olympic champion:* David Epstein, author of *The Sports Gene* (New York: Current, 2013), makes a more modest estimation of the difference between times run on cinder tracks and those run on modern tracks: 1.5 percent.

29 *Edward "Ned" Frederick:* Edward C. Frederick, "In Search of the Asymptote: Projecting the Limits of Human Performance," *International Journal of Sport Biomechanics*, 1986.

31 *But the marathon length:* The idea of an "hour" is also not as rigid a concept as we might like to think, but a full discussion of the fungibility and adaptability of units of time would require another book, and a PhD. To the Romans, an "hour" was roughly one-twelfth of the time between sunrise and sunset.

33 *East Africans win:* Tokyo was added to the World Marathon Majors group in 2012. In 2011, it too was won by a Kenyan.

34 *In 2004, a now-famous:* Dennis M. Bramble and Daniel E. Lieberman, "Endurance Running and the Evolution of *Homo*," *Nature*, 2004, http://www.nature.com/nature/journal/v432/n7015/full/nature03052.html.

35 *This portrait—known as:* Christopher McDougall, *Born to Run* (New York: Knopf, 2009).

35 *A South African scientist named Louis:* Louis Liebenberg, "The Relevance of Persistence Hunting to Human Evolution," *Journal of Human Evolution*, 2008, http://www.academia.edu/5545168/The_relevance_of_persistence_hunting_to_human_evolution.

36 *In his odd and intriguing:* Bernd Heinrich, *Why We Run* (New York: Ecco, 2002).

38 *In 1921, Mallory:* Excerpts from George Mallory taken from Wade Davis, *Into the Silence* (New York: Knopf, 2011).

40 *He is pessimistic:* This article explains Ross Tucker's outlook on the two-hour marathon: http://sportsscientists.com/2013/05/pacing-fatigue-and-the-brain-lessons-from-london.

Chapter Three   **Welcome to Skyland**

45 *The whole country was ripping:* The postelection violence in the Rift Valley was not only about a tricky election. Kikuyu and Kalenjin had long

struggled over the rich, fertile land here. But the political ferment gave the old grudge an extra edge. In all, more than one thousand people died in Kenya's postelection violence before the warring parties struck a deal.

47   *Mutai arrived into a:* Kalenjins take their surname by adapting their father's middle name.

47   *In the first hours:* Mutai's official birthday is October 7, 1981, but since he has no birth certificate, it's hard to know for sure.

48   *This is a sticky topic:* Mutai says that because of his upbringing, he will always feel at home in cold, high, hilly places. He half-jokes that he can't run when it's warm and sunny. When you look at his career, there's some truth to that analysis.

48   *When the British left:* The Masai, a nomadic people, also moved through what is now thought of as Kalenjin country. Eldoret is a Masai name, for instance.

50   *Rakrui and Esther:* The tradition of ear-stretching fell out of Kalenjin culture decades ago.

50   *"He is straight":* Rakrui himself, from whom Geoffrey evidently inherited not only a strong heart but a sedulous work ethic and ticklish disposition, was proud of this reputation as "the Muzungu." It was difficult to talk to him, because of his deafness, and because he spoke no English. So a cousin of Geoffrey's sat between us, with an exercise book and a pencil in his hands, and diligently translated my questions. The cousin then scribbled Rakrui's answers down on a piece of paper for the old man to read, and listened for a response, before translating his replies back to English and telling them to me. It was hard to keep up much repartee in these circumstances, but when I called Rakrui by his nickname, and his grandnephew made the necessary steps not only of translating and transcribing the joke but explaining my goodwill, the old man talked in a language we could both understand. He squeezed my shoulder and laughed himself half to death.

57   *The Kenyan system:* This paradigm of longer events being dominated by athletes who might have had serious careers at shorter distances is being seen throughout the running business. For instance, David Rudisha, the 800m Olympic champion and the world record holder, looks much more like a 400m runner. In fact, although he has only dabbled at the shorter distance, his personal best of 45.13 at 400m is excellent—and

was run at altitude in Nairobi. Rudisha has transferred all that speed and power to the longer distance with great success, and has now run half of the top twenty times ever recorded in the 800m. Likewise, Mo Farah, who is beginning to test his abilities in the marathon, has run an outstanding 1,500m time: 3:28.81—a British and European record. The new generation of distance runners are not pure distance runners. They are turbo-diesels.

59 *Eventually they discovered:* It's surprising how much weight Mutai gives the story of the tea seller and how often he tells it. Despite his many triumphs on the international stage, he seems to believe that his success largely comes down to a decision to drink a cup of tea one dark morning in Eldoret.

Chapter Four   Bright Lights, Big Cities

64 *In 2013, the British runner:* The reported appearance fee for Mo Farah—over two years in which he would run one warm-up half marathon in 2013, with a full-marathon debut in 2014—was £750,000, although nobody from the organization confirmed it. For that sum, he was contracted to run the first half of the 2013 marathon and the full 2014 marathon.

67 *Philippides covered a distance:* Victor J. Matthews, "The Heremerodroi: Ultra Long-Distance Running in Antiquity," *Classical World*, 1974.

67 *After their victory:* Roger Robinson, *Running in Literature* (Halcottsville, NY: Breakaway Books, 2003).

68 *The main financial backer:* John Bryant, *The Marathon Makers* (London: John Blake, 2008).

70 *But people ran "marathons":* Excerpt from Samuel Pepys's diary, http://www.pepysdiary.com/diary/1660/08/10.

70 *"Pedestrianism"—a catchall:* John Cumming, *Runners and Walkers: A Nineteenth Century Sports Chronicle* (Chicago: Regnery Gateway, 1981).

71 *Such races were not:* The purse would be worth around $34,000 in today's money.

71 *The British track historian:* Andy Milroy's article on the history of the marathon, for *Road Racing Stats:* http://www.roadracingstats.com/article_marathonorigins.php.

73 *But in the second half:* There are many odd and fascinating aspects of this unusual period in the sport's history, many related in Brian Phil-

lips's article about nineteenth-century pedestrians for *Grantland*: http://
grantland.com/features/brian-phillips-edward-payson-weston. One of
the strangest is that at some races, the competitors would keep trudging
around the track even when the public had gone home for the night. An
excellent account of the pedestrianism craze can also be found in Nick
Harris, Helen Harris, and Paul Marshall, *A Man in a Hurry* (London:
deCoubertin Books, 2012).

75 *The legend has it:* George R. Matthews, *America's First Olympics: The
St. Louis Games of 1904* (Columbia, MO: University of Missouri Press,
2005).

76 *As John Bryant relates:* Bryant, *The Marathon Makers*.

76 *Tau and Mashiani were:* Floris J. G. Van der Merwe, "Africa's First Encounter with the Olympic Games in 1904," *Journal of Olympic History*, 1999,
http://www.la84foundation.org/SportsLibrary/JOH/JOHv7n3/JOH
v7n3j.pdf.

77 *After 1904, the marathon:* Photographs and narrative of the St. Louis
race posted at "Running Through History," by Jody Sowell of the Missouri History Museum: http://historyhappenshere.org/archives/7266.

77 *They wanted to begin:* Bryant, *The Marathon Makers*.

78 *With these adjustments:* Ibid.

78 *There were 55 starters:* Ibid.

79 *Members of the Irish American:* A similar arrangement continues in
Kenya, where many of the country's best runners are also members of
the police or the army.

79 *This new arrangement:* Bloomingdale's rooftop track no longer exists.

82 *For the next two years:* An account of the Royal Albert Hall indoor
marathon between Pietri and Gardiner: http://life.royalalberthall.com
/2012/02/28/the-first-british-indoor-marathon.

83 *A San Francisco journalist:* Bryant, *The Marathon Makers*.

83 *There was one unusual: New York Times*, 1910: http://query.nytimes
.com/mem/archive-free/pdf?_r=1&res=9F0CE5DE1439E233A25756C
0A9659C946796D6CF.

83 *They ran 13 miles:* Hans Holmer, of West Farms, New York, sometimes
known as "the West Farms Express" and sometimes, confusingly, referred to in contemporary reports as "Canadian," is one of the unsung
heroes of early marathon running. He set a world record outdoors at

"the London distance" at the Powderhall ground in Edinburgh in 1909, in 2 hours, 32 minutes, and 21 seconds, and set another "team" record with Queal in New York, at the shorter distance of 20 miles. Holmer also beat Johnny Hayes at an indoor marathon in Berlin, and George Dunning and Kolehmainen outdoors in a rematch at Powderhall.

85 *In 1968, Dr. Kenneth Cooper:* Kenneth Cooper, *Aerobics* (New York: M. Evans, 1968). A British epidemiologist named Jeremy Morris had laid much of the groundwork for Cooper's book with his seminal papers on the benefit of cardiovascular exercise in the 1940s and 1950s. A review of Morris's contribution to this field is at http://www.bcmj.org/article /exercise-and-heart-review-early-studies-memory-dr-rs-paffenbarger. In his most famous study, Morris compared heart attack disease in bus conductors, who were active, and bus drivers, who were sedentary. The bus conductors were, of course, far healthier. Morris himself died at the age of ninety-nine and a half, in 2009. In a *New York Times* obituary, a fellow scientist—Steven Blair of the University of South Carolina—said that Morris had done "the systematic research that invented the whole field of physical activity epidemiology": http://www.nytimes.com/2009/11/08 /health/research/08morris.html.

85 *Meanwhile, books like:* Jim Fixx, *The Complete Book of Running* (New York: Random House, 1977).

86 *The inaugural New York City Marathon:* Cameron Stracher, *Kings of the Road* (Boston: Houghton Mifflin Harcourt, 2013).

86 *The course for the five-borough race:* Since the first five-borough race in 1976, a few details of the New York course have changed. According to an e-mail between the author and George Hirsch, "In the 1976 race, the course did not run up First Avenue as it does now, but along the path between the FDR Drive and the East River. Fred Lebow immediately realized that there were no spectators and changed it for the second edition in 1977. Also, the first race ran only a few yards around a light pole into the Bronx and then turned back onto the Willis Avenue Bridge. Later, a much larger section in the Bronx was added. Another tweak was made in recent years when the race coming down Fifth Avenue entered Central Park at 102nd Street, up a hill onto the [park's] East Drive. Now the course goes down Fifth until Ninetieth Street, where it enters the park, eliminating the 102nd Street incline."

88 *By its own estimation:* The statistic concerning the New York Marathon's
revenue generation for the city: http://www.marathonguide.com/press
releases/index.cfm?file=NewYorkCityMarathon_110427b.

89 *The inaugural London Marathon:* The route has changed since 1981. The
first London Marathon finished at Constitution Hill, between Green
Park and Buckingham Palace. Between 1982 and 1993, the race was
rerouted slightly so that it would finish on Westminster Bridge. Since
then, however, the marathon has concluded in the glorious setting of
the Mall, directly in front of Buckingham Palace.

90 *In fact, before they:* An account of the Jordache Marathon in *Runner's
World:* http://www.runnersworld.com/rt-miscellaneous/first-professional
-road-race-modern-era?page=single.

92 *Alberto's fortitude was his:* There is a wonderful account of Salazar and
Beardsley's 1982 Boston race in John Brant, *Duel in the Sun* (Emmans,
PA: Rodale Books, 2006).

92 *In 1981, Salazar recruited:* Salazar's Nike deal is reported in Stracher,
Kings of the Road.

94 *Moore remembers the two men:* The exchange between Wolde and Bikila
is contained in this story by Kenny Moore: http://www.kennymoore.us
/kcmarticles/woldehonolulu/woldestory.htm. Wolde was later impris-
oned for nine years by the Ethiopian People's Revolutionary Party.

95 *All fifteen major marathons:* Tokyo was added to the World Marathon
Majors in 2013. It too was won by a Kenyan. The "missing" marathon
is the 2012 New York race, which was canceled because of Hurricane
Sandy.

Chapter Five **Anything Is Possible, Everything Is Possible**

98 *At a certain point in the run:* Mutai says that as a teenager, he used to
ride the train at night from Rongai, where his parents lived, toward
Mumberes, near Equator. He believes the passenger service stopped
after one too many fatal accidents on the line.

100 *Amateur running is an activity:* Average household income of magazine
readers sourced from the Mediamark Research and Intelligence survey,
Spring 2013.

101 *A wind tunnel study:* This calculation about the effectiveness of shield-
ing by pacemakers was made by Alex Hutchinson of *Runner's World,*

and is based on this study by L. G. C. E. Pugh in the *Journal of Physiology*, 1971: http://jp.physoc.org/content/213/2/255.long.

102 *First among them is Berlin:* The world record was broken in Berlin by Paul Tergat in 2003, by Haile Gebrselassie in 2007 and 2008, and by Patrick Makau in 2011.

102 *Athletes will often choose:* There are other factors in who gets invited to races. An Olympic or world champion is attractive, whatever his or her personal best. And Haile Gebrselassie will keep getting invited to races until he is a hundred years old, because he is one of the few true stars the marathon has, and he knows how to talk to reporters.

103 *It was a dazzling move:* The splits from Mutai's two runs at Eindhoven were provided by Edgar de Veer.

104 *Throughout his time as a professional runner:* Those who watched Haile throughout his career used the schoolbook arm as a "tell" to understand when he was struggling in a race. When Haile was tiring, the imaginary schoolbooks would get bigger and heavier.

106 *In fact, Haile made:* This handpicking of rivals is not uncommon among top marathoners. Geoffrey Mutai himself asked that Patrick Makau not be invited to Berlin in 2012.

107 *In 2003, Tergat raced:* It was after this world record that Tergat claimed the two-hour marathon was "impossible"—but that time might "chide" him.

108 *With the help of Sean:* Hartnett had designed similar maps for Tergat, but Hartnett remembers Haile being much more invested in their importance.

108 *In the 1920s and 1930s:* Runners before Nurmi had also deduced that a flat pace was an efficient way to run, even if the Finn was the first to talk about it in detail. In 1835, Henry Stannard won the ten-mile one-hour challenge on Long Island by keeping to a steady pace set by a rider on horseback.

112 *It now belongs to Tadese:* It is one of the sport's most puzzling conundrums that Zersenay Tadese of Eritrea has never run a single marathon in a competitive time. He has been the fastest half marathoner for years, with three sub-59 finishes and the world record at the distance, but his personal best in the marathon (at the time of writing) is only 2:10:41, set in London in 2012.

117 *After the race, the little Ethiopian wept:* Federico Rosa witnessed Kebede's tears himself, and the story gained currency in Kenya. Gatheru, Wanjiru's best friend, told the story of the race many times himself, but attributed Sammy's staying power to what he said was a Kikuyu fondness for money. (He was a Kikuyu himself.) There was simply no way Sammy would pass up the opportunity to win half a million dollars. Gatheru then told me an off-color joke that he said Kikuyus often tell against themselves: that the only way a doctor knows whether a Kikuyu is dead is to drop a bag of money by the bed, and to see whether his patient sits up.

Chapter Six   **Kids, That Was Real**

126 *Steve Prefontaine, the tragically:* The article featuring the comments of Ron Clarke and Steve Prefontaine in *Sports Illustrated:* http://si.com /vault/article/magazine/MAG1087086/index.htm.

126 *Back at his training camp:* Claudio Berardelli remembers Sammy Wanjiru trying the same thing in training. While the rest of his colleagues attempted to keep a steady, fast pace, Sammy would tear ahead of them, or lag behind before trying to rip past them. He was getting his body ready for race day.

127 *Mutai remembers his fellow:* In 2014, the East Africans racing at the Boston Marathon made the mistake that Mutai would not permit them to make in 2011. Meb Keflezighi, the American marathoner who won the 2009 New York City Marathon, made a surge that nobody in the pack covered. Meb then got into a good rhythm, and opened up a huge gap. By the time the East Africans reacted, it was too late. Meb won the race. In terms of personal best, there was no way he should have won. His best time was five minutes slower than the fastest Kenyan's. He was also thirty-eight years old. But the East African contenders made a tactical error, and lost because of it.

130 *Mutai was a rich man:* Mutai's management, Volare, was unwilling to disclose his earnings. Meanwhile, shoe contracts and appearance fees— the two most lucrative income streams for a top marathoner—are not publicly available. However, based on conversations with other managers and athletes, as well as public information about prize money and time bonuses, it's possible to arrive at a rough estimate of Mutai's wealth.

130 *Mutai had the money:* This belief that the best athletes should live a holistic and self-sufficient life while in training camp is strongly held. At the Global Sports camp in Kaptagat, where Geoffrey Kamworor and Emmanuel Mutai are based, the athletes divide chores between them, and report to an athlete "chairman" who solves any domestic niggles. There are dozens of similar camps across running country.

135 *What's more, he had:* New York also pays substantially bigger appearance fees than Berlin—although Mutai has always maintained that he looks for success first, and that "money comes after."

136 *Only four men before him:* Bill Rodgers did the Boston–New York double twice, in 1978 and 1979. The other doublers were Alberto Salazar, Rodgers Rop, and Joseph Chebet. Chebet's double, in 1999, was particularly sweet. The previous year, he had finished in second place in both races, each time by a margin of only three seconds—in Boston to Moses Tanui, and in New York to John Kagwe.

138 *In his outstanding book:* Epstein, *The Sports Gene.*

140 *Since the publication:* In general terms barefoot "form"—running, as if barefoot, with a lighter tread, and a mid- or front-foot strike—is widely considered healthier. In the barefoot form argument, cushioned shoes are deemed to encourage athletes to run badly. This observation becomes moot, however, when one is talking about Kenyan runners, all of whom grew up running barefoot, and who mostly have excellent technique before they first wear sneakers.

140 *In any case, what:* The debate about barefoot running is also crucial in terms of understanding the preeminence of East African runners. At the time of writing, Yannis Pitsiladis and several other scientists were preparing to publish new data that proved what Pitsiladis himself had long believed: that kids who grow up running in bare feet develop with better "foot health"—stronger, more responsive feet and ankles—than their shod counterparts in Kenya and in other countries. This might be one factor to explain Kenyan running dominance. By the time "habitually barefoot" kids start running in sneakers, in their teens, their tendons and muscles are already well developed, their bone strength is superb, and they are less likely to have problem arches in their feet. Their form, meanwhile, is rock solid. As a follow-on from this discovery, Pitsiladis told me it would be interesting to see whether a runner

might ultimately develop stronger if he trained without shoes, for longer, before switching to sneakers.

141 *A University of Calgary:* The University of Calgary study on the performance of Boost foam: http://www.tandfonline.com/doi/abs/10.1080/19 424280.2013.799566?journalCode=tfws20#.UlaASVC388A.

142 *What Mutai seemed:* Despite being a widely held belief in Kenya, the simplistic understanding of energy sources coming from "fats" and "sugars" is challenged by the science. Greg Whyte, a leading British sports scientist, dismisses this bifurcation of energy sources as profoundly misleading. Energy production, he says, does not switch gear in a race—it all comes from ATP—but as heat rises in an athlete's body, the process becomes much less efficient later in a race. It may be that great athletes like Mutai were somehow able to be less inefficient later in a race.

Chapter Seven   Not Everyone Can Run Like Geoffrey Mutai

148 *An average young rural:* Many Kalenjin kids look painfully thin, but a low body mass index (or BMI) connected to an energetic lifestyle is, according to a recent study, one factor behind the Kalenjin running phenomenon. Pitsiladis and Lieberman concluded, "The highly active and energy-demanding lifestyle of rural Kenyan adolescents may account for their exceptional aerobic fitness and collectively prime them for later training and athletic success." http://www.ncbi.nlm.nih.gov/pmc/articles/PMC3689839.

148 *The question is not:* A study that discusses this phenomenon about altitude living and training: F. C. Cerny, J. A. Dempsey, and W. G. Reddan, in the *Journal of Clinical Investigation,* 1971, http://www.jci.org/articles/view/107497.

148 *As David Epstein explains:* Epstein, *The Sports Gene.*

149 *"A helpful combination":* Haile Gebrselassie would identify himself as an Oromo, but one morning over breakfast before the 2013 Berlin Marathon, we were discussing Epstein's book, and specifically the analysis of the Oromo and Amhara cited within it. Haile told me a little-known fact about his family. Some of his ancestors, he said, moved from the Amhara region "one hundred and fifty years ago" and he has a significant portion of Amhara ancestry in his DNA. Ancestry isn't everything when it comes to distance running.

155   *At its best, this system:* If a European agent does screw his African charges
out of money, or sleep them a dozen to a hotel room, it is because he has
recognized an uncomfortable truth about Kenyan and Ethiopian distance runners. Even in big races, featuring world champions or record
holders, the promoters of big marathons struggle to market their elite
African runners as personalities. And if you're just another fast African, you become somewhat expendable. No agent would treat a runner
badly if he knew there was not another to take his place. (Dodgy agents
are nothing new, either. Dorando Pietri's brother Ulpiano, who managed the Italian marathoner in the running craze of 1908–1910, had
him running marathons almost every fortnight. He also took 50 percent
of his winnings: a usurious relationship.)

159   *As far as explaining:* In 2014, Tucker and others were attempting to shine
a light in that forest by testing elite Kenyan runners at their laboratory
in South Africa, but the conclusions of those studies were months away
at the time of writing.

159   *For instance, as Tucker:* Dr. Michael Joyner notes that most studies
in the area of "trainability" have been testing responses to "low dos-
age" training, rather than the high-intensity schedule undertaken by
elite athletes. If you took a large population and exposed them to elite
marathon training, "who the hell knows what would happen?" (Joyner's
contention is that "most young men" are capable of running sub-three
hours for the marathon, given the right training.)

160   *Upon Rotich's return to Kenya:* John Manners, "Kenya's Running Tribe,"
Sports Historian, 1997, http://library.la84.org/SportsLibrary/Sports
Historian/1997/sh172d.pdf.

162   *To make his point:* Waquie also murdered Joyner, who came "about fif-
teenth" in the race.

163   *His old Ethiopian rival:* When I saw Kebede win at the 2012 Chicago
Marathon, the thought occurred to me that perhaps we believe the par-
adigmatic Kalenjin runner's body is the perfect shape because Kalenjins
win a lot of races, rather than the other way around. If tiny guys like
Kebede kept winning races, then maybe we'd reassess.

164   *In Japan, to use one:* A report on the increasing tallness of Japanese
schoolboys: http://www.nytimes.com/2001/02/01/world/tokyo-journal
-the-japanese-it-seems-are-outgrowing-japan.html.

164 *Clearly, there is something:* The increase in average height reflected the improving diet and lifestyle of Japanese children, and the elimination of once-deadly infectious diseases. This is unsurprising given the trauma the country suffered during World War II, and its subsequent economic boom. One theory also contends that the trend for bigger Japanese children seems to be connected to the modern Japanese trend of sitting on chairs, rather than sitting on the floor.

164 *Nobody on earth:* Alun G. Williams and Jonathan P. Folland, "Similarity of Polygenic Profiles Limits the Potential for Elite Human Physical Performance," *Journal of Physiology*, 2008, http://jp.physoc.org/content/586/1/113.

165 *What's been most interesting:* Denis Noble, *The Music of Life* (Oxford, UK: Oxford University Press, 2008).

165 *John Manners, the American:* Some Kalenjin maintain this practice. Julius Arile was a cattle rustler from West Pokot, whose weapon of choice was an AK-47 assault rifle. He is now a professional marathon runner with a 2:12 personal best, and was in contention until late in the 2013 New York City Marathon.

166 *It is not hard to imagine:* Manners, "Kenya's Running Tribe."

166 *According to one history:* From the 1997 essay "Why Kenya?" by Toby Tanser: http://www.kenyarunners.com/pages/167371/page167371.html ?refresh=1112199340095.

Chapter Eight   Only with Blood

173 *A recent study:* An article featuring the study on EPO benefits in *Runner's World:* http://www.runnersworld.com/elite-runners/study-kenyans-get-performance-boost-from-epo.

173 *In the Tour de France:* In *The Secret Race*, by Tyler Hamilton and Daniel Coyle (New York: Bantam, 2012), Lance Armstrong's former teammate described how "Edgar" (their nickname for EPO—a play on Edgar Allan Poe) was used to boost their hematocrit levels after an extended period of exertion.

174 *But not many Kenyans:* Of the fourteen Kenyan men and women who were given bans for doping in 2012 and 2013, only two tested positive for EPO. One Ethiopian was also banned for EPO.

175 *Often it was an athlete:* Berardelli once had to visit a hospital to see an

athlete who had been found in bed with another man's wife. The cuck-olded husband beat the runner to a pulp.

176 *This is when:* If this part of Kisorio's testimony is true (and there is no particular reason to suspect otherwise), then he ran a sub-59 half mara-thon clean.

177 *Kisorio told Hajo Seppelt:* An English-language article on Hajo Seppelt's investigation, in *Athletics Illustrated:* http://athleticsillustrated.com /interviews/hajo-seppelt-kenyan-doping-exposed.

180 *Several doping cases:* The German documentary had fingered the world record holder, Patrick Makau, as being a client of one of these phar-macies, using the somewhat flimsy evidence that his picture was on the wall, and that the owner of the store said he was a "client." Both Makau and Zane Branson, Makau's manager, categorically denied the charges. In a statement, Makau said: "The story falsely associates me with a particular retail store (located in the Hilton Hotel, Nairobi) and claims that I am a direct customer. This is not correct. I have never been on the premises. The only thing in that shop that suggests that I have anything to do with the store is an old national newspaper clipping with my photo, taped to the wall, together with many other clippings of other athletes' races. . . . I will be racing with a clear conscience."

182 *While some of the top:* Alberto Salazar's full remarks to the Duke confer-ence are available here: http://law.duke.edu/sportscenter/salazar.pdf.

183 *In 2013, a long investigation:* The *Wall Street Journal* investigation of Salazar's athletes and the prevalence of hypothyroidism in the group: http://online.wsj.com/news/articles/SB1000142412788732355060457 8412913149043072.

183 *In 2011, Shorter gave:* Shorter was quoted in *Runner's World:* http:// www.runnersworld.com/rt-miscellaneous/1981-cascade-run-race -changed-sport?page=single.

185 *In 2013, the Canadian:* The WADA report: https://www.wada-ama.org /en/resources/world-anti-doping-program/lack-of-effectiveness-of -testing-programs.

Chapter Nine   He Kills Everybody

189 *There was loose talk:* A few coaches had seen Mutai get drunk in the aftermath of the World Cross Country Championships in 2011, but

most seemed to think that when he was in deep training, he was dry.

193   *Dave Bedford, the impresario:* Bedford's courting of Geoffrey Mutai had started more than a year earlier. He attempted to secure Mutai's presence at the race in 2012, but was thwarted by the Boston Marathon officials, who were naturally keen that their record-breaking champion return to defend the title he won in 2011. Bedford and Mutai's management made a deal that he would appear in London in 2013 instead.

194   *But, for those few seconds:* Before the 2013 New York City Marathon, the sporting apparel company Asics ran a promotion in which they invited people off the street to see how long they could maintain Ryan Hall's 4:46-per-mile marathon pace on a treadmill. The answer in most cases was seconds, rather than minutes.

195   *The pacemakers were cajoled:* After the race, Kipsang said that he spoke to Emmanuel on several occasions saying, "Let us just relax the pace," but that this advice only served as encouragement to Emmanuel, who kept the speed high.

195   *Still, eight competitors:* There were nine men on this pace, if you included Mo Farah, who finished his day's work at halfway.

195   *After the halfway:* Between 20km and 25km, Emmanuel Mutai and a small group ran a 14:30 split, which is 1:59:28 marathon pace.

196   *Meanwhile, as Wilson:* Kipsang later conceded that his preparation for the London Marathon had not been perfect, and that his shape was only "ninety percent."

199   *They began the race:* Kipsang's halfway split in Berlin was 40 seconds quicker than Geoffrey Mutai's the previous year.

201   *In Frankfurt, in 2011:* When he returned from that race to Iten, I asked him about his feelings on missing the world record by such a small margin. He thought about the question for a long while, before saying, "It is possible to feel two things."

Chapter Ten   **Broken Stones**

207   *Long before Mutai:* It's likely Mutai's children will never experience the same feeling. They do not need to walk to school, or work a farm. In their free time, they play in their manicured garden with their toys. If and when they get jobs, they will be professionals—working in offices. Neither of Mutai's daughters, brought up in a rich part of a bustling

town, speaks Mutai's mother tongue, Kipsigis, a language for poor people from the countryside. They speak Swahili, and English. It's a source both of pride and regret for Mutai, who is now teaching them the rudiments of Kipsigis.

209 *Everybody had forgotten:* One of the factors that helped Hermens achieve this landmark was a mixtape he made, filled with one hour of his favorite motivational music, which was pumped out on the stadium's speakers. Hermens hasn't retained a full copy of the playlist, but he remembers the cassette tape started slow with Rod Stewart's "Sailing" and finished with Bruce Springsteen's "Born to Run."

209 *But he was a student:* The record was first set by the great English runner Alf Shrubb in 1904, in Glasgow. Shrubb ran 18,742m in an hour.

209 *Haile shattered the:* At the time of publication, Haile had also set five Masters (over-40s) world records.

210 *Instead of setting:* Several studies have found that elite runners perform best at very cool temperatures: http://www.runnersworld.com/races /whats-the-optimal-temperature-for-marathons.

210 *But it's possible elite:* A *Runner's World* article on circadian rhythms: http:// www.runnersworld.com/race-training/the-physiology-of-morning -v-evening-workouts.

212 *As David Hannah, the former director:* Toni Reavis passed on that line by David Hannah.

Postscript

219 *On December 17, 2014:* Scott Douglas, "Sub-2:00 Marathon Project Launches," *Runner's World*, December 17, 2014, http://www.runnersworld .com/elite-runners/sub-200-marathon-project-launches.

About the Author

ED CAESAR has contributed to the *New Yorker*, the *New York Times Magazine*, the *Atlantic*, *Outside*, and *Smithsonian*, among many others, and has reported from a wide variety of locations, including Iran, the Democratic Republic of Congo, and Kosovo. He is the winner of nine journalism awards, including the Foreign Press Association of London's Journalist of the Year for 2014. He lives in Manchester, England. *Two Hours* is his first book.